Introduction to Natural Healing

Letting your Body Heal Itself

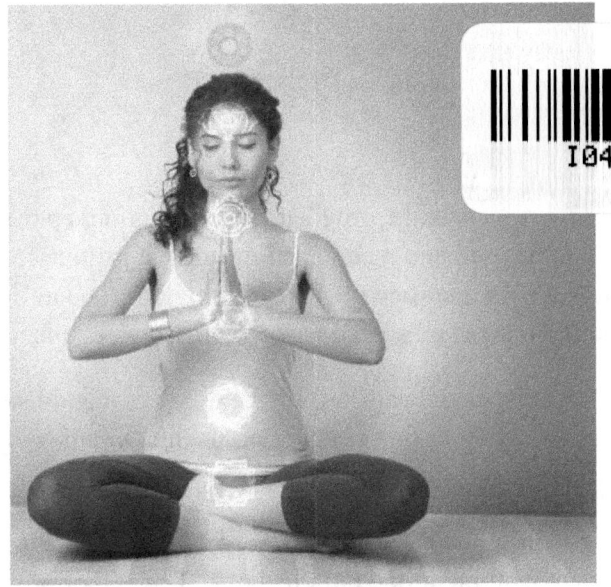

I0411949

Healthy Living Series

Dueep Jyot Singh

Mendon Cottage Books

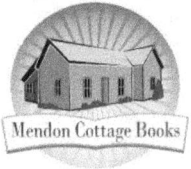

JD-Biz Publishing

Disclaimer

The information is this book is provided for informational purposes only. It is not intended to be used and medical advice or a substitute for proper medical treatment by a qualified health care provider. The information is believed to be accurate as presented based on research by the author.

The contents have not been evaluated by the U.S. Food and Drug Administration or any other Government or Health Organization and the contents in this book are not to be used to treat cure or prevent disease.

The author or publisher is not responsible for the use or safety of any diet, procedure or treatment mentioned in this book. The author or publisher is not responsible for errors or omissions that may exist.

Warning

The Book is for informational purposes only and before taking on any diet, treatment or medical procedure, it is recommended to consult with your primary health care provider.

Our books are available at

1. Amazon.com
2. Barnes and Noble
3. Itunes
4. Kobo
5. Smashwords
6. Google Play Books

Table of Contents

Introduction to Natural Healing 1

Letting your Body Heal Itself 1

Introduction 4

Principles of Natural Healing 10

Earth 15

Massages 15

Massaging Process 19

Mud Therapy 25

Mud Baths 28

Water 32

Hydrotherapy 35

Hip Baths 38

Steam Baths 39

Hot Foot Baths 41

Hot Water Fomentation 43

Air 45

Sunlight 49

Ether 54

Knowing More about "Fasting" 54

Difference between Fasting and Starving Yourself Deliberately 57

Conclusion 63

Author Bio 65

Publisher 76

Introduction

Why are more people all over the world looking towards natural cures and natural alternate methods of medicine in order to cure themselves? The day of fast drug-induced cures and relief is slowly fading and giving weight to alternative medicines and therapies in order to cure the body.

These ancient remedies and therapies have been in existence all over the world for millenniums. The ancients swore by them but then they did not have powerful drugs, having a detrimental effect on their biochemical system. That was the time when they believed in not overloading their systems with pills, drugs and medicines, which supposedly cured them of their body's ills.

Thanks to this dependency since childhood on medicines, because we see our elders eating them by the handful, is it a wonder that a number of us have lost the capacity of getting cured naturally? Much before powerful drugs came onto the scene, Mother Nature was already providing her living creations with excellent rejuvenating and healing systems which would replenish the wounded and damaged cells with healthier tissue and heal the body on its own.

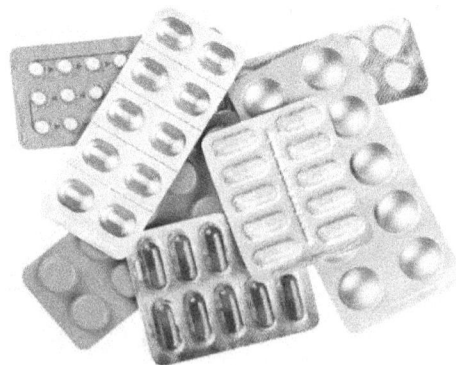

Most of us are chronic pill poppers, eating all these powerful medicines without rhyme or reason, just because the doctor said so.

Left on its own, Mother Nature is the most powerful doctor known in the universe. However, man has been supplementing her curative powers with natural herbs which aid in the healing process for millenniums.

Naturopathy is one of these ancient healing systems, which use a number of natural therapies in order to heal the body in the most beneficial and long-lasting manner.

Naturopathy does not use any chemicals or any medical preparations. If any herbs are to be used, they are going to be hundred percent natural. These therapies are not going to give you an overnight cure. Unfortunately, these overnight cures are the side effects of powerful chemical drugs. But you do not know that these cures have masked the symptoms of the disease from being visibly apparent.

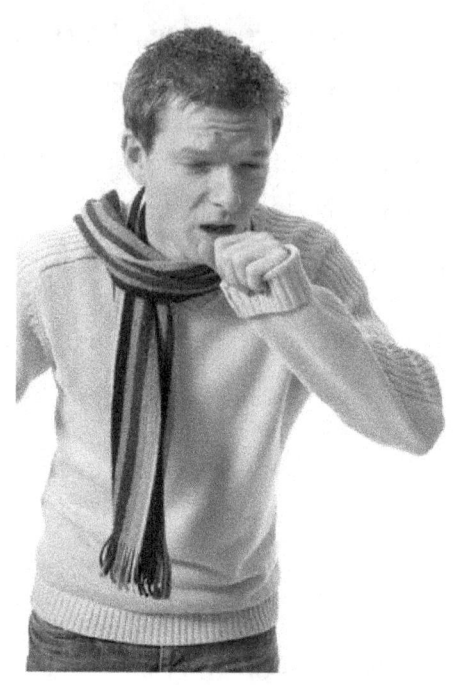

If you find yourself in such a situation, what is your first reaction? You make a beeline for the nearest medicine cabinet or your favorite over the counter remedies drugstore/pharmacy. And then you swallow whatever they give you because they promised to get rid of your cold miraculously, overnight.

You wake up in the morning, after having swallowed a powerful pill at night, supposedly able to get rid of that cold overnight. Hey, you feel wonderful. Your nose is not clogged up. You do not feel congestion in your system. That is just wonderful.

You think yourself cured.

Unfortunately, that pill gives you just temporary relief. The infection in your body is still there somewhere inside. It has not had a chance to clear itself naturally. But you have must be symptoms with a powerful medicine which is preventing Nature from doing her work.

The effects of these temporary relief drugs are going to wear out within a given time limit. And then you pop another pill, which is going to give you surcease from coughing, sneezing and sniffing for the next 8 hours.

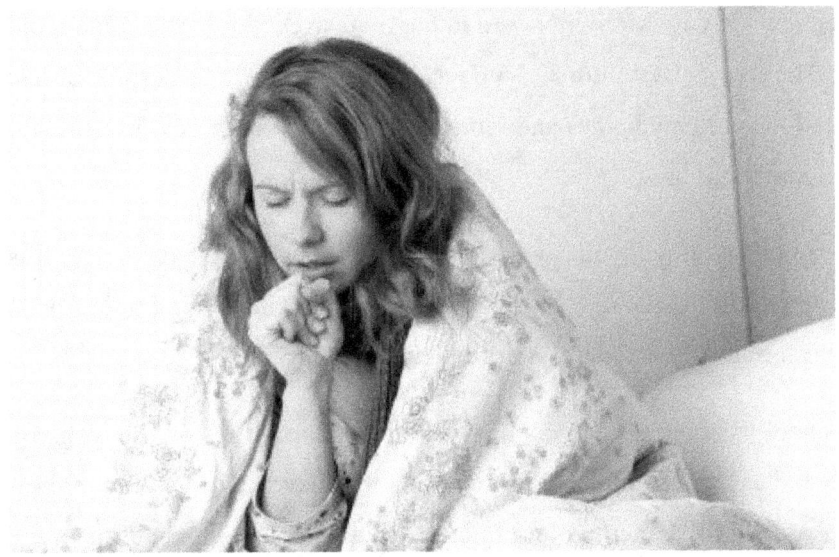

The problem with all these drugs is that, apart from weakening your own natural immunity system, they are going to have some harmful side effects. You may find yourself cured of your cold, but you may find yourself suffering from tummy ailments and headaches.

You may think them to be the aftermath of your cold. In fact, they are the side effects and aftermath of all those powerful drugs you have been taking.

So you go back to your doctor. He recommends some more drugs to counter the side effects of the previous drugs he had recommended to you oh, say, a week ago. So you take them, supposedly to cure the side effects. So now you are caught in the vicious Catch-22 situation.

You have just finished recovering from cough and cold. You end up with tummy problems and headaches and a weak immunity system, possibly leaving your body vulnerable to even more future infections.

How much better it would have been if you had just allowed yourself to be cured naturally by Mother Nature in her own sweet time. The cold would have run its course within 3 to 5 days. You are going to be surprised to see that all the cold medicines and remedies available out there ask you to take medicine for 5 days.

When you are cured, you say, hey, that was because of the medicine. It is just wonderful, is not it. You do not know that the incubation time from start to finish of a cold is 5 days in normal circumstances!

This book is going to tell you all about how natural ways of allowing your body to heal itself without resort to medicines have held sway for thousands of years. All these methods are time-tested and have been the basis of alternative sources of medicine in ancient civilizations down the ages.

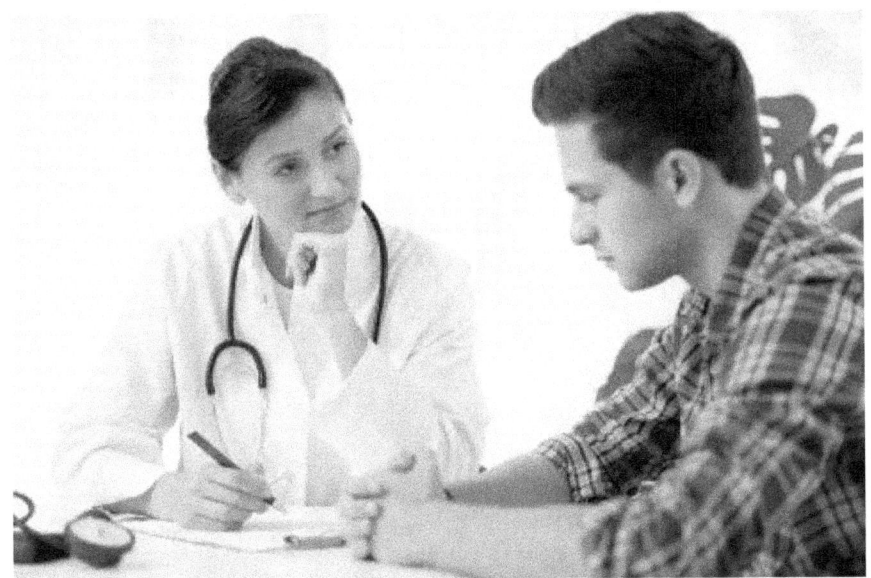

Have you been eating your medicines regularly? [Unfortunately, a number of us have the tendency to run to a doctor for instant remedies at the tiniest hint of a sniffle.]

Principles of Natural Healing

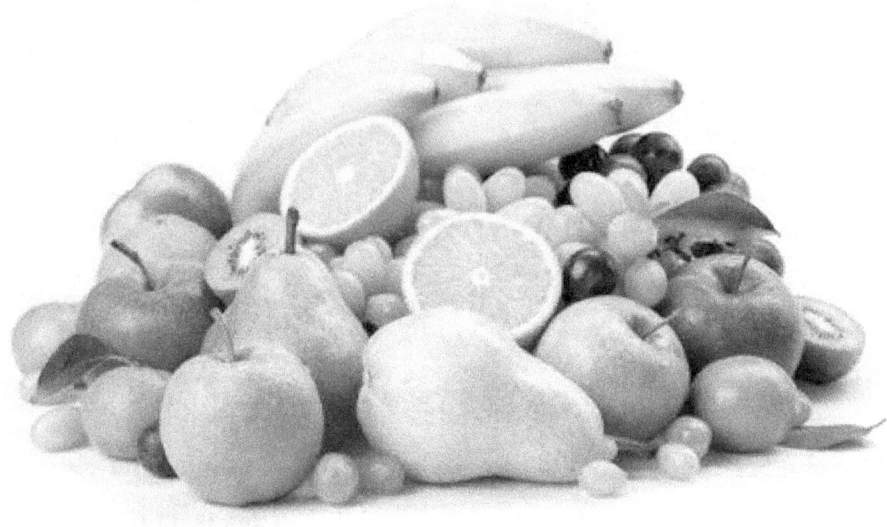

Healthy natural foods are an integral part of your body healing itself on its own.

Naturopathy practitioners believe that the body's self-healing characteristic is one of the most powerful gifts given to it by nature. Even though many diehards may scoff at this alternative medicine practice, which may not be encouraged in their own lands and dismissed as quackery – believe it or not, there are some places out there where herbs and ancient remedies are still considered to be heathenish medicines not fit for civilized and educated people; this is, of course, propaganda promoted by pharmaceutical companies want to sell their own possibly potentially harmful drugs and do not want to encourage alternative sources of healing – who is to stop you from looking at an alternative source of health, which has been practiced down the ages by healthy and long-lived people?

Natural remedies and healing practices are to cure ailments which are lifestyle induced. Nobody bothered about cancer and other tobacco related problems in Europe in medieval times, until the time when Sir Walter Raleigh and his fellow Elizabethan explorers brought tobacco back to England from the lands they had explored. So smoking became a part and parcel of the European lifestyle. That also brought with it diseases related to nicotine, – also known as the good weed.

In those days, medical practices in Europe were primitive and not very advanced. However, there were medical practitioners in the shape of wise women, barbers, and nuns who knew all about herbal remedies through knowledge and experimentation. But they did not practice the cures openly because you needed just one hysterical woman to shriek, she is a witch and the wisdom of the ages would burn with a Wise Woman on the stake.

So, in that day of superstition and darkness, women kept their family remedies to themselves. They never allowed other people to learn about the knowledge passed to them from their foremothers. In fact, any woman who managed to raise a full family through good food and cleanliness would be considered to be a witch. However, if one or more of her kids died due to sickness, brought about by her carelessness, and bad food, she was one of the common throng and would never have anything to fear from the flames.

Is it a wonder, then, that the practice of mumbo-jumbo, spells, black magic and other superstitious ideas were encouraged by quacks and self-styled powerful shamans, witch doctors and other such people all over the world down the ages? This was the prerogative of just one person in the tribe. In many parts of the world, you went to him to invoke the gods on your behalf and take your medicine, literally and figuratively.

The ones who were really serious about their art healed their patients with natural remedies wrapped up in chants, songs, dances and other acts of showmanship.

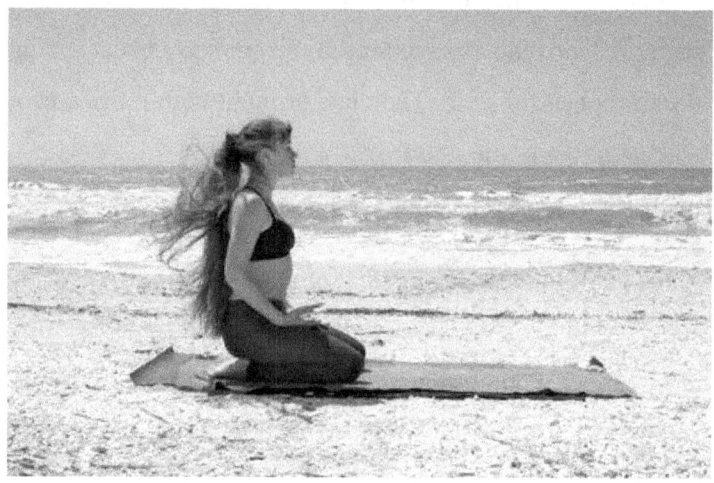

Naturopathy is just one part of the natural healing systems being practiced down the ages. These systems include Chinese medicine, Ayurveda, Yoga, homeopathy, Siddha and the Greek, Egyptian and Persian ancient medicine systems.

Saint Luke was a great physician before he became an apostle. He was a Greek who went to Egypt to study medicine, after having learned all he could from his Greek teachers. He also studied the medical systems of the civilized nations of those times. All this medical lore was available to just a select few, and return on papyri and scrolls and were deemed very precious.

A majority of the knowledge wealth of the ages has somehow now been lost to us. However, some alternative medicine practices are universal throughout the world, like a naturopathy therapy.

Naturopaths believe that 99% of the diseases caused in the human body are due to the violation of natural laws. This includes lack of self-discipline ignorance, and overindulgence in food and drink. Naturopathic therapies are going to reduce or undo those resulting ills.

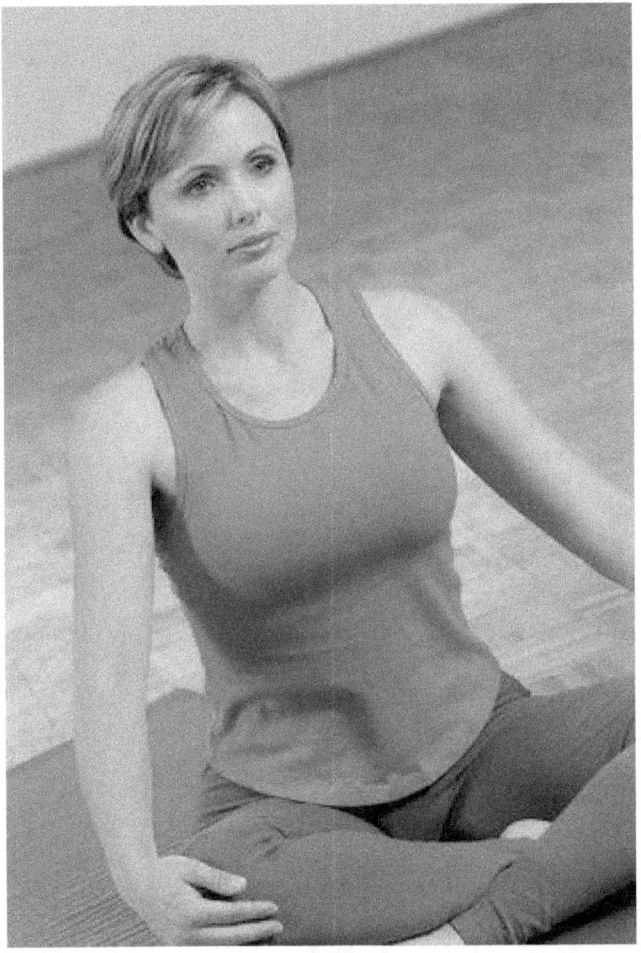

Naturopathic treatments include a number of elements which are part of the cure.

So we begin with the elements needed for the body to heal itself naturally.

Earth

Mother earth is one of the most important elements which are going to help cure you. Elements of earth, including mud baths and mud packs are going to rid you of skin diseases and chronic gastric ailments.

Massage is also an important part of this element.

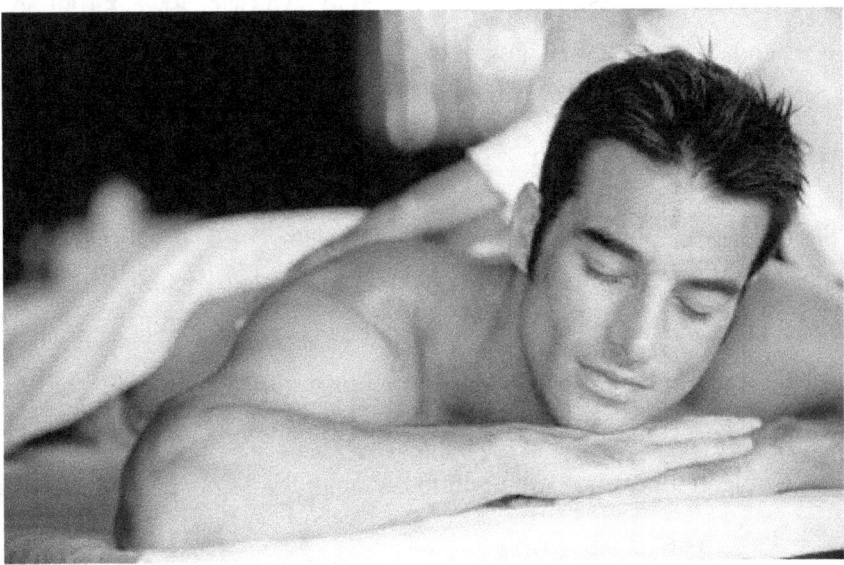

Healing massages have not only been a part of relaxation down the ages, but they also help in physiotherapy and tissue rejuvenation and growth.

Massages

The art of massage has been known since ancient times, all over the world. This is an integral part of naturopathic treatments. This procedure was used her particularly for thousands of years in Greece, Rome, Egypt, China, and in other parts of the world where medicine was considered to be an evolved science.

A proper massage is going to have a very beneficial and salubrious effect on your external and internal organs. The moment you find yourself being treated to massage, the muscles of the skin "tone and wake up", and the pores open up. This is due to the better circulation of the blood throughout the system. This means that all the toxic poisons in your body are getting eliminated in a natural manner.

In many parts of the East, this massage used to be a twice a week routine to keep you healthy, and every day, in order to get rid of specific problems. However, nowadays with so many people bothered about time constraints, massage has become a luxury.

I remember as a child being given a head massage by my uncle. The word shampoo comes from it. It is called champi. Uncle slathered his hands with lots of coconut oil, and then gave my poor head, scalp, and hair a brisk massage for about half an hour. Of course I protested, because this was a very unusual procedure, and I could not understand why anybody would want to subject himself to being pummeled with the palms of 2 hands, in an oil shampoo.

But he said that it would keep my scalp problem free. I got off after half an hour, rather easily, because he said that was enough, while my younger brother had to go through one hour of a massage shampoo. I still remember the tingling sensation in my scalp, and the funny sort of feeling in my head. But those were the cells waking up and taking notice.

And then when he told me that children were massaged every day, down the ages by their grandmothers and other elders of the family so that their muscles grew strong and well-toned and their limbs grew straight, I could only give grateful thanks that father had not ordered our nanny to massage her charges every day. Even though I could see her eyeing us longingly, because according to her we were not being brought up in the traditional manner!

That is the reason why the people of that area had beautiful skins, well-toned muscles, straight limbs, plenty of energy, and continued this through their whole lives. This was the best detoxification procedure for them.

Massages also reduced the tension in the muscles after a hard day's work in the fields or on the training grounds of a battlefield.

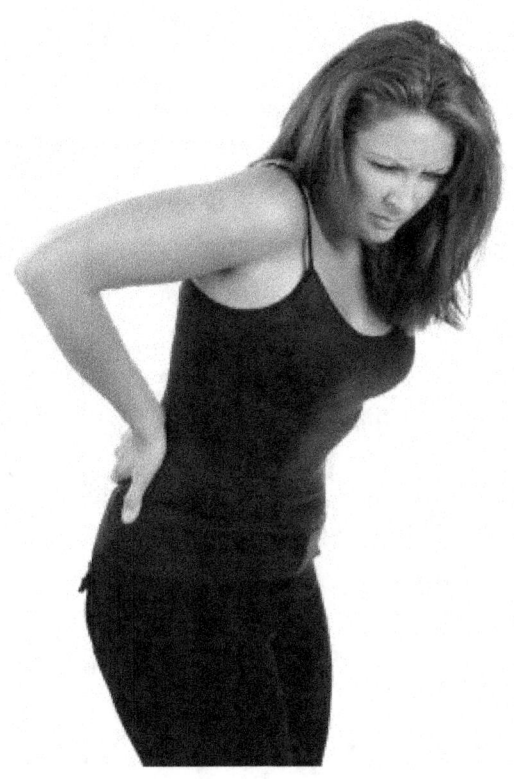

A proper and regular massage on the affected area can help relieve local pains.

Gentle massages relieve muscular pain. I remember an old wise woman massaging my shoulder, because she wanted to strengthen the muscles there. I had a tendency of putting the shoulder joint out, ever so often as a child. Thanks to that massage procedure, I have never had my shoulder joint coming out of its socket, ever again.

Massages also improve the circulation of the blood. If you feel lots of cold, especially in the winter, it means that you need to massage that area gently to get the blood flowing. That means that particular part of your body is going to be augmented with more nutrients. This improves the healing power of that particular area.

You may want to read Kipling's Rewards and Fairies, where an Elizabethan wise woman Dame Whitgift managed to get her injured nephew on his feet again, by massaging him thoroughly with her chosen herbs for 6 months. You can call this a forerunner of physiotherapy to heal the body.

That is why in ancient times, people who knew how to do massage properly were very well thought of in their tribe. A slow and gentle massage with just a light pressure on top of your skin surface is going to relax the nerves. A vigorous massage at that same time is going to stimulate lax and possibly injured nerves and increase their potential and efficacy.

In the same manner, you can promote the activity of your digestive system and your urinary system by massaging the abdominal region. Your powers of resistance are also going to benefit by this massage, because the liver is going to function efficiently.

So how do you go about massage?

Massaging Process

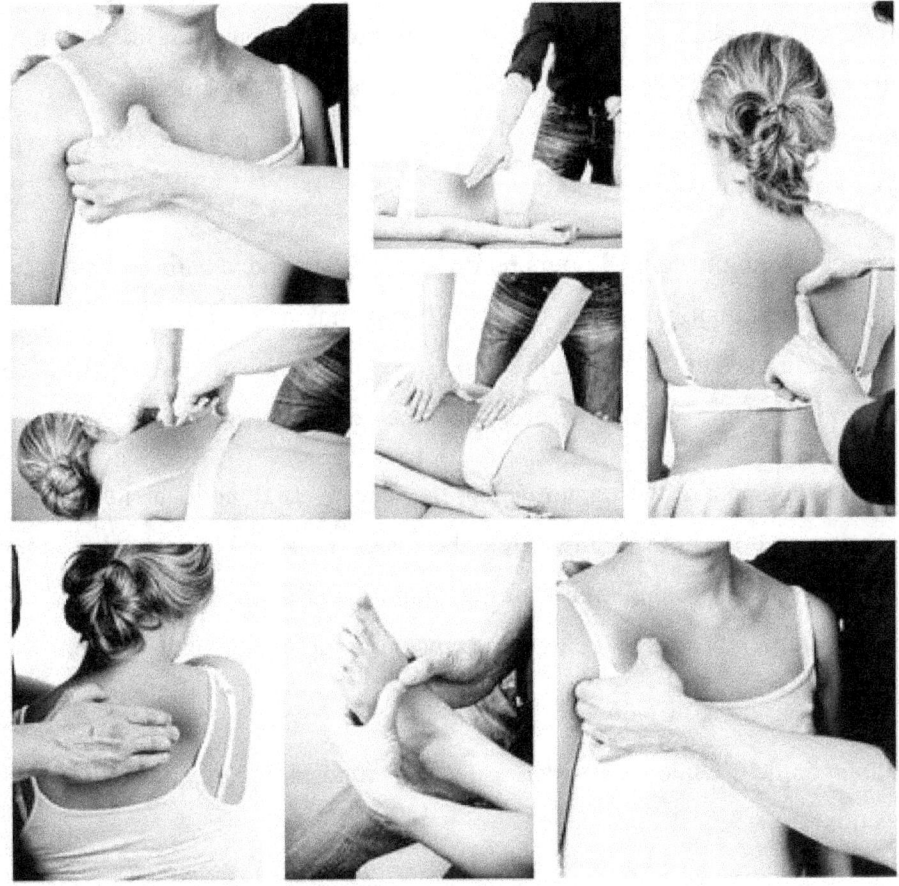

If you intend to do the massage yourself, remember one thing – the movement **should be towards the heart**. That is the way massage has been done traditionally, except when you are suffering from fever, skin diseases, or when you are expecting a child. In the latter case, you are not going to massage the abdomen. This abdominal massage is also not going to be given if you suffer from gastric problems, ulcers, or any stomach ailments.

Traditionally, dry palms were used for massage, but healers normally like using soothing oil, especially if the skin is very dry, or the body is weak.

I normally prefer a soothing oil like almond oil, olive oil or wheat germ oil for normal massages. For massages to heal, I use a stronger oil like coconut oil or mustard oil. Remember the latter oil is rather strong smelling and powerful and that is why it is always used to heal damaged tissue or to keep your body healthy.

This massaging is done 4 hours before you need to take a bath on a sunny day. It takes about half an hour for a full body massage. After that bake yourself in the sun for 20 minutes. And then take a shower without using any soap. Sesame oil is considered to be the best oil for healing massages.

This is why most of the senatorial and patrician work done in ancient Rome was always done in the baths. While the slaves massaged the patricians, they did their relaxing and talking about O tempora, O Mores. Discussions of times and morals are still being done when a group meets to relax, even 2000 years down the line.

Some people use talcum powder, especially in hospitals, to reduce the friction.[1]

---

[1] Way back in the 90s I noticed this being done at my brother's hospital by the nurses and asked them not to do that, because that clogged up the skin pores. Instead, I asked them to do the massaging to prevent bed sores or during therapeutic treatments with almond oil.

Believe it or not, the rapidly healing patients consider this to be a luxury, and went back home and broadcast the news that our hospital gave full value for money where real honest to goodness "Badam Rogan" was used for massaging![1] We did not know much about olive oil, then. But olive oil is also an extremely good massaging oil, if you go by the "Greek Gods" physique of all those who live in the Mediterranean region.

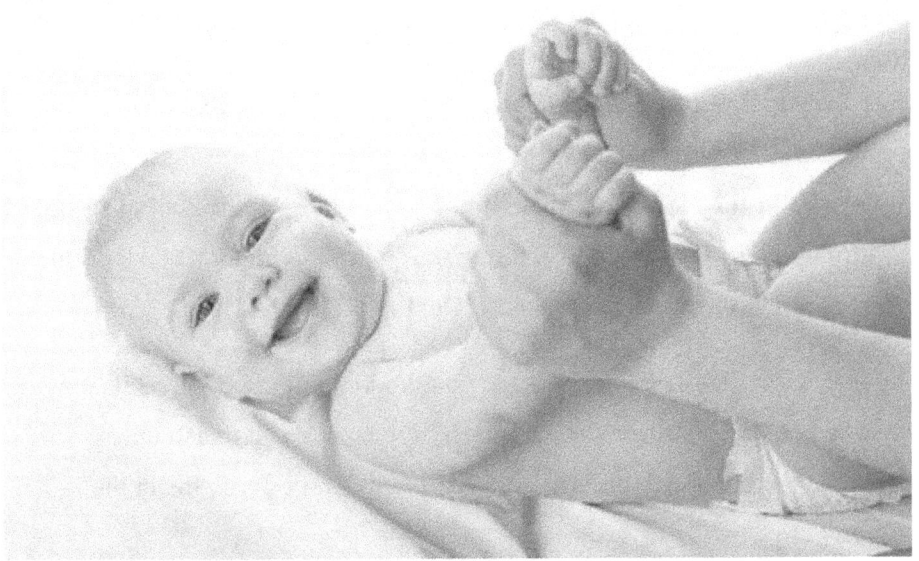

Mom giving baby a massage before his bath is good fun!

Important tip before you start the massaging process yourself. If you are suffering from high blood pressure, your massaging movements are going to be reversed from those given below. You are going to start from head to foot, instead of from foot towards head.

The normal or healing massaging process is going to begin with the proper massage of the arms and the legs. **Remember that the movement always has to be towards the heart.** Begin from your pulse points in your arms, and move towards your shoulders. Massage that area as often as you want.

If they had their loving nonnas around when they were children, they must have been massaged thoroughly with olive oil.

Then, you are going to start from the feet, moving up the limbs towards your stomach and loins region. That is part 2 of the massage process.

Part 3 is an important one – when you are going to massage the area around your heart. The movements around your heart region in the chest must **always be in the clockwise direction. That means you are going to start at 12 o'clock of the clock face. After that go to 3 o'clock, then 6 o'clock, the 9 o'clock and then back to 12 o'clock.**

After that, you are going to massage your abdominal region. Do this only if you are not suffering from any stomach problems like stomach upset, appendicitis, duodenal or gastric ulcers, or any sort of growths in the tummy.

The massage direction – phase 4 of the massage – is going to be in the anticlockwise direction. **That means you are going to start at 12 o'clock of the clock face, then you are going to 9 o'clock, then 6 o'clock, then 3 o'clock, then back to 12 o'clock!**

Phase 5 of your massage process is going to be massaging your back. This is rather enjoyable, because you are going to be using a towel. Here, hold the sides of the "bunched and stretched" towel in both your hands and do vigorous movements from shoulder to mid arm and back again in to and fro motions. This is in the upper back region. Then comes the lower back which you are going to massage up and down with the cloth – phase 6.

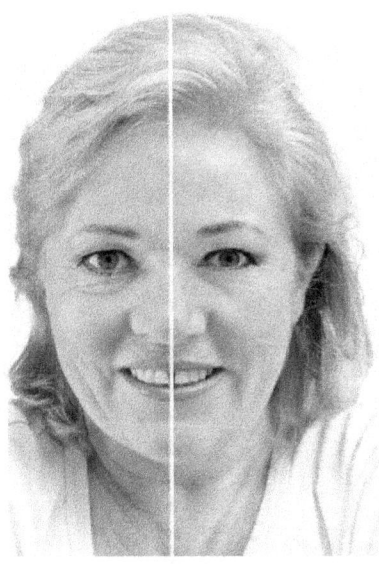

Antiaging creams can hide your wrinkles temporarily because they have moisturized and plumped out your skin. Thus they give you the illusion of youthfulness. I would rather you massage your face with natural traditional products like honey and milk cream.

The 7th phase is your face, and head region. I would suggest asking an experienced beautician, to teach you how to massage your face, especially if you are a woman and are bothered about wrinkles. But remember that the massage direction should always be towards the heart. Personally I never touch my face at all, – except when washing with warm water and no soap or chemical creams – and that means I never bother about wrinkles or fine lines.

They are part of the aging process, and I am not going to speed up that process by subjecting the skin to chemicals or antiaging creams which need me to massage the skin morning, noon and night. Nothing doing. My natural moisturizer is honey and milk, mixed together so that the honey does not go sticking all around the place.

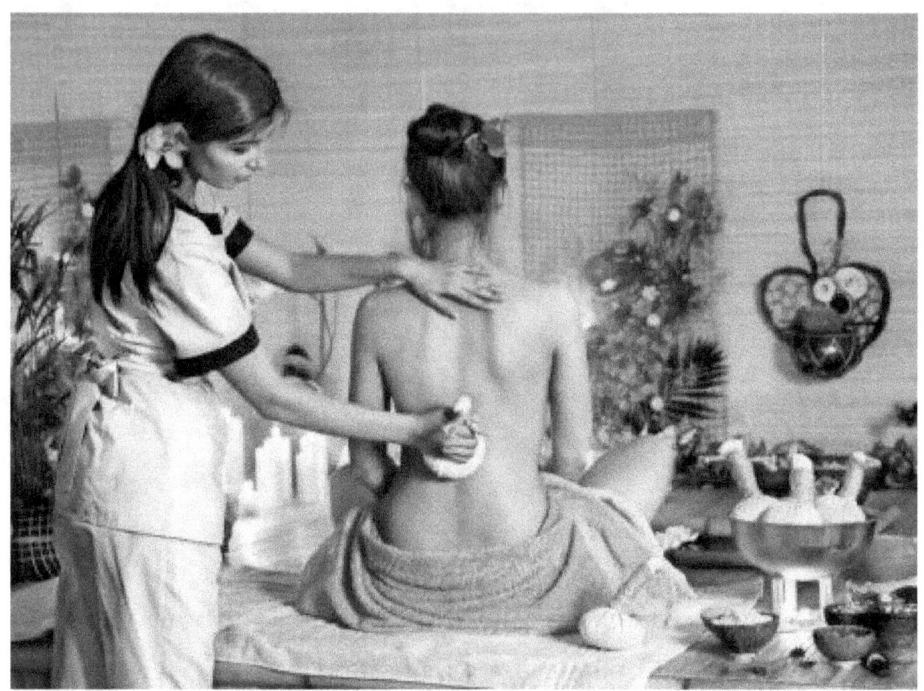

A massage should be followed with a lukewarm water bath. Cold water is what the ancients advocated, but later on it was found that even in the summer, fresh water was lukewarm-ish, especially when it had been heated with the rays of the sun in the afternoons. So use that fresh water in the afternoon to have a nice invigorating shower. Scrub with a loofah.

Mud Therapy

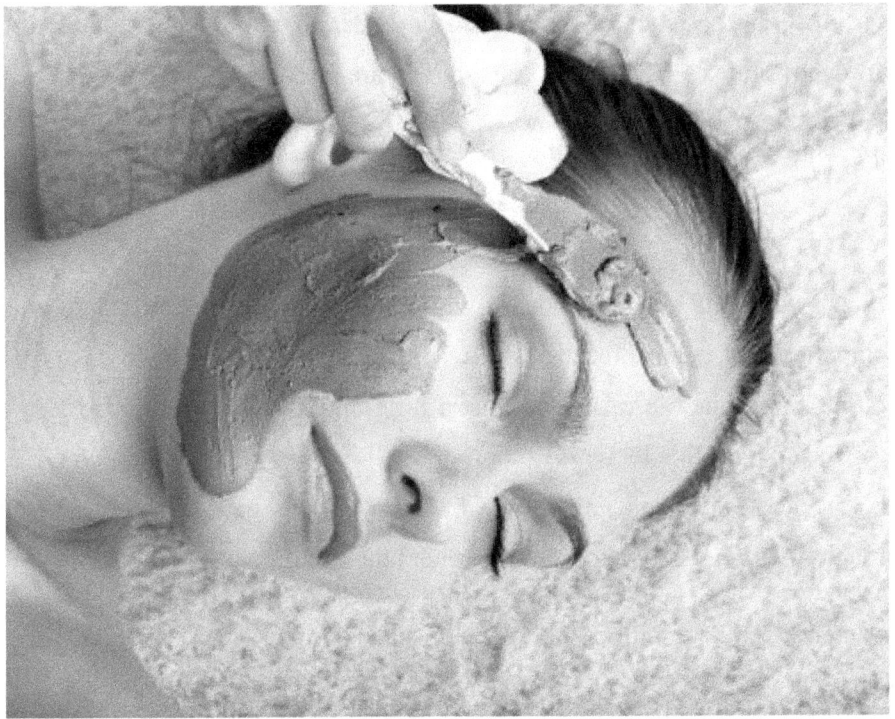

Mud and clay has been used down the ages and all over the world, not only as a beauty aid but also to prevent and cure skin diseases.

For many people the idea of mud therapy or a mud bath is something which they are going to come across only in an expensive spa. But in natural cure systems, mud therapy and clay therapy has been an accepted way of helping heal the body naturally.

This is one of the best external healing and therapeutic agents benefiting mankind.

Can I use any sort of clay, you may ask?

Actually, the clay used by Native American natural healers was rich in calcium. It was called Calcium Montmorillonite by geologists. Apart from that, different varieties of clay, like Bentonite, Rhassoul, [this comes from Morocco] Fuller's Earth, and French green are also used in clay therapy.

You can find these easily in the USA, from

https://www.mountainroseherbs.com/#AID=130283

Fuller's earth has long been known in the East as one of the most important components of beauty facemasks. It is also used to draw out toxins. After you make a paste out of it, with just a little bit of water, just spread it over an affected part, like let us say a boil or anything septic. You can also spread it on a piece of cotton muslin and bandage it. It is going to draw out the infection within a couple of days, and heal the tissue.

I remember my grandmother telling me all about warfare in olden times. When the Warriors went to the battlefield and got injured, their warrior women went to the nearest source of water – the river, got out a handful of river mud and slapped it on the warrior's body to heal the wound.

I had a feeling that this would infect the wound, because anything inside the wound would have remained there, with no way to get out. But she told me that the wounds were cleaned of dirt, grime and dried blood with a mixture of honey and water. Now that was sensible, I thought, and the ancients really knew about the healing power of mud and clay.

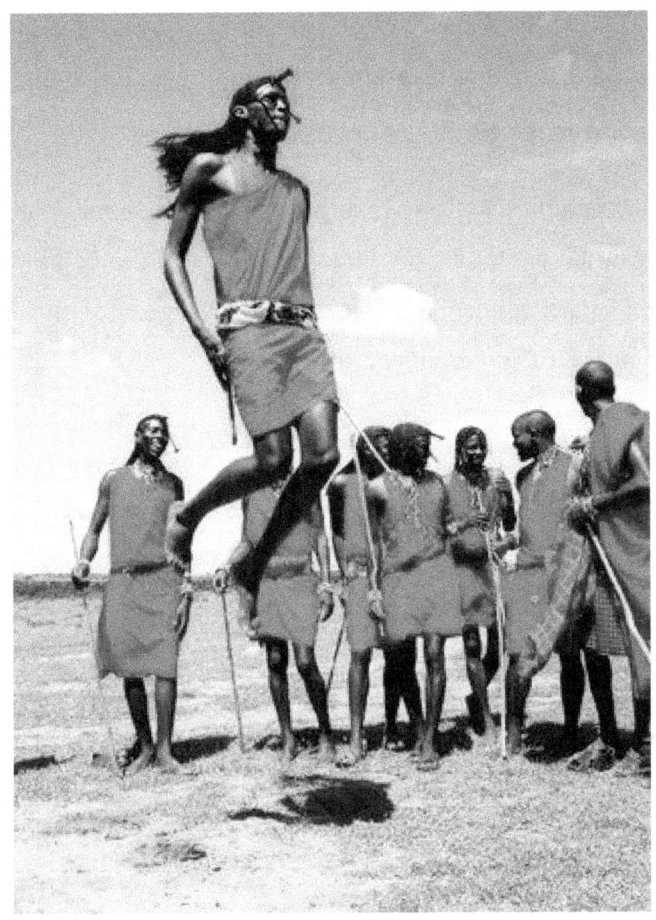

This proud Masai "Moran's" ancestor would have not bothered about injuries much, except for plugging that injured region with river mud or clay.

The lion hunting Warriors, the Masai have been known to casually slap some mud taken from a clean source on their injuries, incurred during a lion hunt.

Being of a practical nature, my immediate reaction was, but they were scratched by the claws of a lion, and that was definitely full of material which would cause infection and possible poisoning. I was told that they dipped themselves in the river first and got rid of the blood. Well, that means the wound was cleansed before the mud pack was slipped on with mud collected from the bottom of the river.

This clay is generally used as a mud paste. It can be applied directly on to the body, or in the form of a poultice. Usually, you are going to be treated with this mud pack applied on that particular region of the body which exhibits symptoms of any ailment or disorder.

Mud Baths

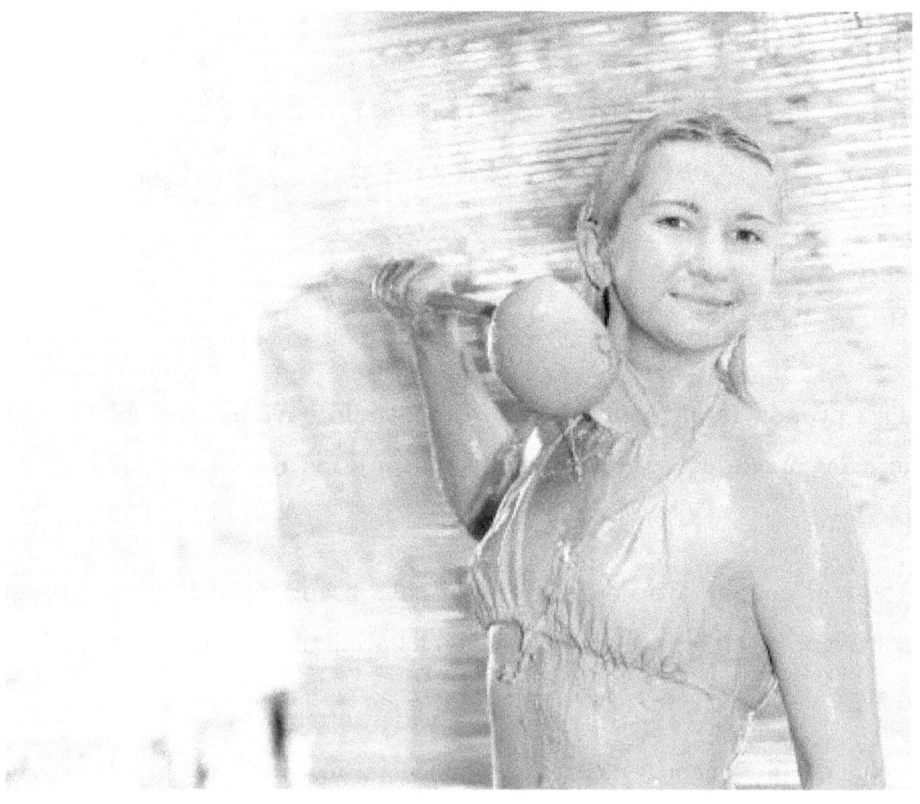

During a mud bath, mud or clay of a suitable consistency is generally applied over the whole body and you can lie in it with your head outside.

Clay of any color can be used for a mud bath, as long as it is free from toxins, chemicals and harmful materials. If the clay is viscous, a bit of sand is also mixed with it. The clay is going to be sieved , so that any stones, coarse materials and pebbles do not interfere with your mud bath experience. This clay is then going to be dried out in the sun.

When you are getting ready to apply the clay on your body, you need to mix it with a little bit of water and make a paste. Spread it all over your body. If you want to apply it only on some particular part of the body, it is going to help cool the tissue during the healing process. If you cover it with a thick cotton or woolen cloth, this mud bath is good for healing.

If you want to reduce the body's temperature, leave the clay uncovered.

Mud baths were normally given to people suffering from fever by the ancients, to reduce the body's temperature and to help heal it. After half an hour or an hour depending on the severity of the ailment, the mud was removed. The Treatment could be repeated, in case the patient did not seem to show any drop in temperature.

When you are using this therapy to treat a feverish body to cool it, you need to wipe clean the body with a piece of cloth to remove the mud. After that you need to bring it to normal temperature by rubbing all that area with your palms.

If this mud bath has been used to warm the body, remember to wipe clean the dried mud with a cloth which has been **wrung in cold water.**

Clay and mud therapy has been in use for millenniums to help cure fevers, diarrhea, stomach problems, constipation, and other such internal disorders. This is going to afford immediate relief from localized pain, especially when you are suffering from stomach problems.

I have seen that this is really efficient, especially for reducing swellings. A sprain in the ankle in the shape of a Clay pack applied to that swollen area, 2 times a day reduced the swelling considerably. You can consider this to be some sort of natural fomentation, but I was cooling the injured tissue.

Clay absorbs all the toxins in your body. So if you have any sort of infection, especially something suppurating, try applying a Clay pack on it. It is going to absorb all the poisons. It is also going to heal your ailment, without leaving any scars.[2]

---

[2] I found this site pretty amusing reading and very informative.

http://prettywitchy.com/the-purifying-benefits-of-mud-and-how-to-use-healing-clays-for-health-and-beauty/

Please remember that I am definitely not endorsing any of these sites or products! This is just for your benefit.

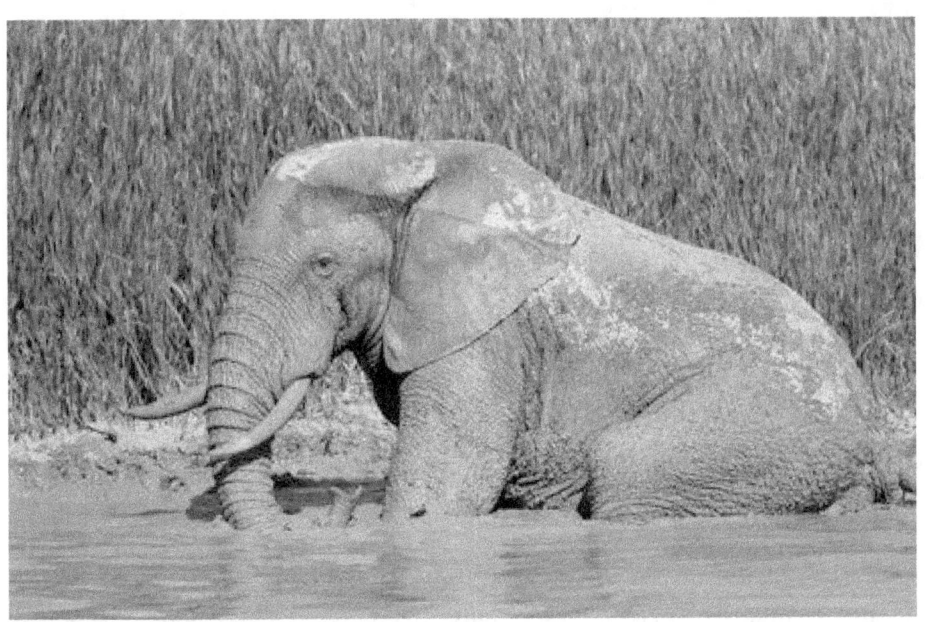

Water

Water is the 2nd element, which is going to help your body heal itself naturally. Naturopaths swear by water therapy. Water therapy is known as hydrotherapy in their circles. Not only is it an excellent stimulant, but it is also capable of reducing fever, a good antioxidant, and tones up your system considerably.

But before I tell you more about water therapy, I would like to give you some ancient tips with which you can gain full benefits from water. Of course you are not going to drink water, which is muddy, has impurities in it or is from an open source outside like a river, or a pond. Any stagnant water should definitely be avoided, especially if you are on a hike and come across an open water source.

But hey, you are dying of thirst, and you need to drink some water. If you see life forms in it, and the water is flowing, you can take a chance of drinking it. But if it is still and stagnant, you are better off trying to look for another water source.

If the water is not pure, boil it and filter it. That is going to get rid of a major part of the impurities. Do not drink too hot or too cold water. We have this nice habit of going straight to the refrigerator and chugging straight from the bottle. Not only is this terrible for our teeth, but doing this, when you are overheated, coming straight in the house from a terribly hot, sweltering summer outside, and there you are, you have opened yourself up to a bad summer cold and associated problems.

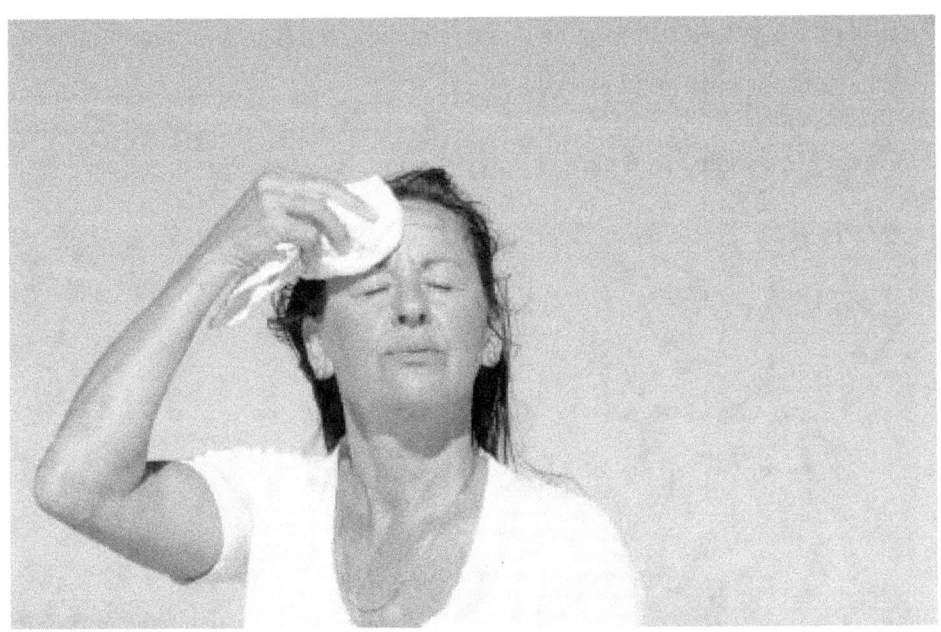

Dehydration and loss of water, especially in the summer are one of the main causes of heatstroke and summer ailments.

Believe it or not, many of the brands of the expensive mineral water which you buy in bottles off the supermarket shelves are often not as pure as they are advertised. In fact, once I managed to get into one of these factories where this water was being "manufactured!". It was then bottled as pure mineral water and sent all over the world under a very famous Brand Name.[3]

Here are the ways in which you can keep yourself healthy, just by drinking water. Drink four large glasses full of water, first thing in the morning on an empty stomach. The ancients normally recommended anywhere between

---

[3] Name Withheld. It is a multibillion-dollar industry. And I do not want them to screech libel.

half a liter to 1 L of water on an empty stomach, but that is a bit too much for me and for you, in the initial stages.

Drinking less than 5 to 6 glasses a day is going to lead to constipation.

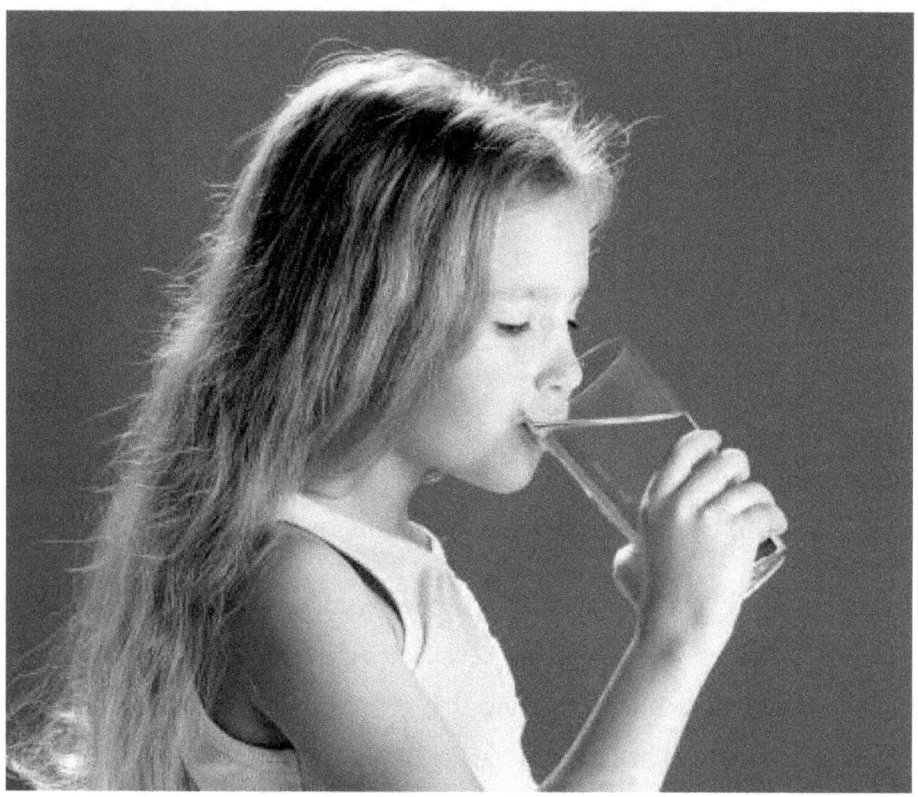

Aaah, precious water...

You can increase the intake of water early in the morning, as time goes by. This is normally done without you Brushing your teeth, washing your face, or doing your early morning ablutions.

This water is going to be placed at your bedside at night. Traditionally, it was placed in a copper utensil, so that it could absorb all the qualities of that metal throughout the night.

After you have drunk the water, you can go ahead with washing your face, brushing your teeth, showering, shaving, and so on. But do not eat or drink anything for one hour after you have drunk this water.

This water is cleansing your body of the toxins accumulated during the nighttime. It is also going to stop you from suffering from constipation.

Do not drink any water when you are eating your meals. If you have to drink anything liquid, you may take a couple of mouthfuls before or during your meal, or half an hour before a meal. But the ancients did not drink anything for 2 hours until after a meal, so that the saliva and the gastric juices could do their best work. The water that you drink during the meal is going to interfere with the gastric juices produced in your body during the digestion process.

You can also control your weight by drinking the juice of one lemon, and one tablespoonful of honey, in lukewarm water first thing in the morning. This is also excellent for your skin, keeping it well moisturized.

Hydrotherapy

Different hydrotherapy processes include steam baths, hot foot baths, enemas, hip baths, fomentation, and irrigation of the stomach. Many of these procedures are still being used in spas, while others are considered to be old-fashioned and obsolete – including enemas, hip and Foot baths.

Naturopathy advocates regular bathing. Gone are the days when the idea of "bathing harms the skin" was spread in many parts of the world, especially in medieval times. At that time, body odor was masked with sweet smelling perfumes.[4]

Naturopathy includes keeping your body clean through regular bathing. Not only does this wash away all the dirt, but the scrubbing process stimulates circulation and relieves fatigue.

People who perspire freely should bathe twice a day. Lukewarm water or cold water is best for bathing purposes. Hot water bath may be very pleasant, but they take away the precious moisture from your skin. On the other hand, a cold water bath is very stimulating because it boosts up the circulation.

---

[4] It is said that Princess Caroline of Brunswick – in keeping with the times – had such a displeasing body odor that her other fastidious husband, the future George IV, [notorious as Prinny and having learned to keep clean in body and clothing from his friend Beau Brummell] had said, "we may have married that woman, for the sake of England, but being near her is a punishment. "

She also did not like him much. So she encouraged that attitude by not changing her outer or inner garments for 6 months at a time. They did manage to have one child, Princess Charlotte, but it is well known that his wedding night was the only time when George came near his "legally wedded wife" for the sake of the throne of England.

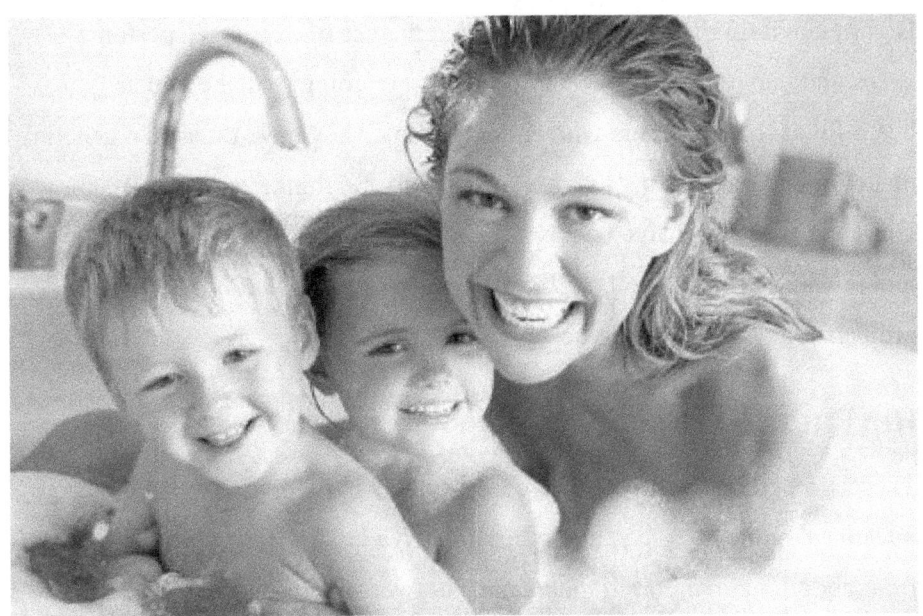

My grandmother, come summer, come winter used to get up at dawn and take a cold water bath. That was what she had been taught by her elders. We spoiled little brats definitely shuddered at the mere thought of a cold water bath, every day, including the coldest winter.

Funnily enough, she never caught a cold, even though we thought cold and pneumonia would have been the aftermaths of taking cold water baths when it is snowing outside. But then, I believe, a very strong immunity system, and a body accustomed since childhood to a cold water bath allowed her to be so stoic.

She never used soap while bathing, but used natural cleansing remedies like Clay, milk cream, oatmeal and wheat bran as cleansing agents. These are the cleansing remedies which are still being used in many parts of the East, where expensive beauty creams, powders, lotions and "lip reddeners" are still considered to be taboo to "good girls of good family!"

Do not entertain the mistaken notion that the use of expensive perfume soaps and very expensive beauty products are going to make you as beautiful as the superstars who endorse them. They have their own genetic make-up and so do you. Both are miles apart. So thinking that cleansing your skin with expensive beauty products is going to keep you young looking, and healthy, well, that is all a multibillion-dollar industry's propaganda working overtime.

Hip Baths

These are extremely effective to cure ailments in the liver, stomach, intestines, kidneys, spleen and other digestive organs. If you are suffering from abdominal pain or cramps, take a hot water hip bath. Place a napkin which has been dipped in cold water on your head and scalp during this time.

You can alternate between a hot water and cold water hip bath after spending 2 minutes in each tub to gain even more benefits of this natural curing process.

A hip bath has a very special type of tub. It is about 30 inches long and 20 inches wide. It is also known as a sitz bath because the patient sitz in it, no pun intended, immersed to his hips.

This URL can give you some more information about hip baths.

http://www.wisegeekhealth.com/what-is-a-hip-bath.htm

So alright, I did not bother to buy a hip bath. I just went to the nearest caterers and asked them whether they could sell me a round metal/plastic tub in which they collected used plates, cutlery and crockery after the feasting was done.

They had plenty of them, exactly right for what I wanted. I could "accordion" myself into that tub with my knees outside, and the upper portion of my torso nice and dry.

So once you have your bathtub installed, fill it up with lukewarm water to a depth of 8 – 10 inches [up to 25 cm.] Now drink a glass of warm water and sit in the tub, with your abdomen and parts of your thighs submerged in the water. The upper trunk portion and the legs are going to be outside your tub.

Keep massaging the abdominal region with a little bit of pressure, using a coarse and thick towel.

A hot water hip bath in the winter should take about 15 minutes. In the summer, you can enjoy a cold water hip bath for about half an hour.

Make sure that you dry yourself completely after a hip bath. You are going to take it on an empty stomach. Do not eat anything for about one hour after you have taken this bath. Let nature do her own curing.

Steam Baths

These baths in the form of steam boxes began to be more well-known and popular in the Victorian era, when spas started introducing them in mountain resorts for tourists. However, they were universally known to eliminate toxins from the body for thousands of years. In fact, this was a known method in which the ancient Romans brought down their weight with an increase of the metabolic rate of their bodies.

In ancient Rome, steam baths were made through pipelines of boiling hot water hitting ice cold water of the bath and everybody boiling himself in the ensuing steam. Nowadays, specially designed cabinets or steam boxes are used in steam baths. They are rather expensive, so spas which use them regularly prefer investing in such boxes. And that is what you enjoy during your sauna bath in that spa.

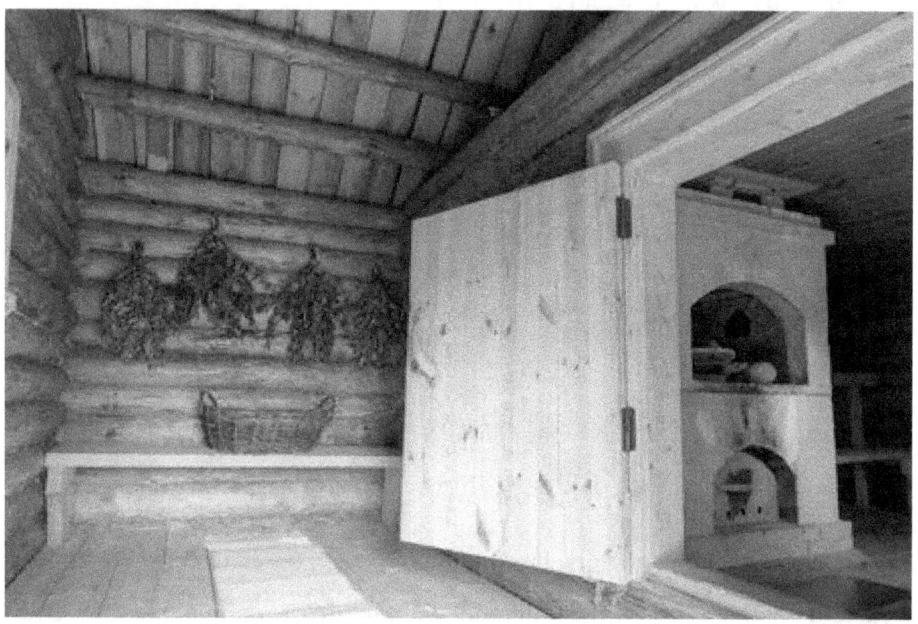

Traditional sauna baths have birch brooms or brooms of other herbs to apply on your body during the scrubbing process.

This bath is taken when the stomach is empty. Drink a glass of warm water and enter the cabinet with minimal clothing. Apply a towel dipped in cold water around your head to keep it cool. After all, matters are going to steam up in a while.

This is normally done under the supervision of an attendant, who keeps sprinkling cold water on your head to keep it cool.

Steam from either a steam pipe or from any other steam source is let into the cabinet. If you find yourself getting lightheaded or dizzy, come out of the steam bath immediately.

When sufficient perspiration has been formed, – 10 to 15 minutes, – get out of the steam bath and take a cold bath immediately. Your body is going to feel young and rejuvenated.

Do not take this steam bath, if you are a heart patient, are expecting or have high blood pressure.

If you are a DIY sort of person, this URL may prove interesting, especially when it is so easy to make.

http://www.instructables.com/id/Steam-bath/

Hot Foot Baths

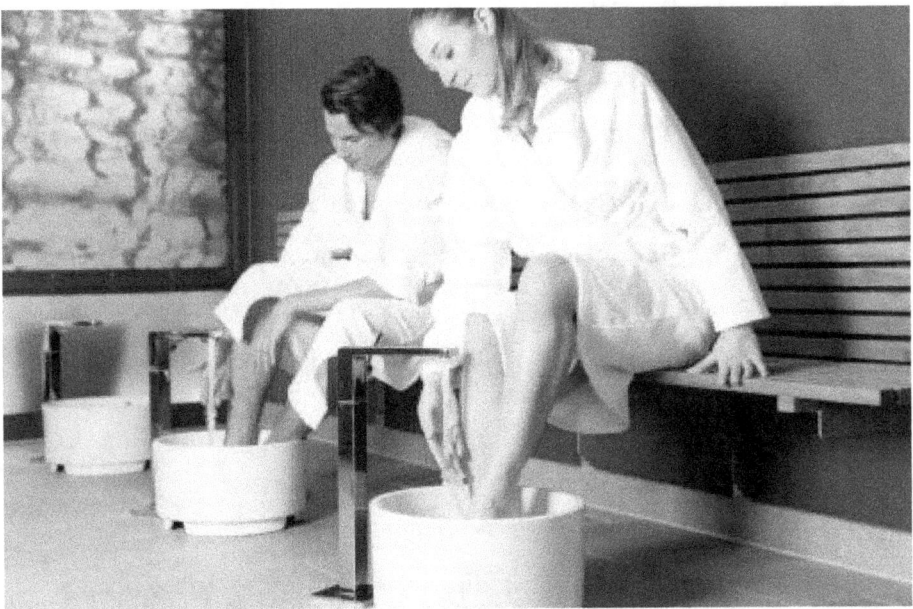

This is extremely easy to set up, to reduce congestion of water in your upper torso. You are going to use fairly hot water in a bucket. Fill the bucket up, about three quarters, and pick up a woolen blanket.

Now place the bucket in front of a chair, sit down and wrap the blanket around you. Have a napkin dipped in cold water ready at hand to place on your head.

Immerse both feet at the same time. You are going to start perspiring within the next 15 to 20 minutes. When you have totally sweated it out, literally and figuratively and find yourself drenched with sweat stop your bath immediately. Make sure that you keep your head cool by sprinkling cold water on the napkin on top of your head.

Ladies should make sure that their hair is dry and unconditioned, when taking this bath. Wet, half dry and just shampooed hair is going to help you to catch a cold, really quickly.

After you have finished bathing, wipe your body with a cold, wet cloth. Then lie down for 10 minutes.

So your legs are all red. That is because the circulation in that particular area has increased. Your feet are going to reach their normal state of color and tan in about half an hour. Unless, of course you are Superman and plunged your feet into boiling hot water and allowed them to cook. That is when you need the help of a doctor.

If you have not managed to bring up a sweat in the next 15 to 20 minutes, that means the temperature is less. Take out your feet, and add 4 glasses of boiling water into the bucket. Then dip your feet in and wrap the blanket again around you.

Your blood pressure is going to decrease during this procedure. That is why you need to lie down because you are going to feel all dizzy and weak.

That is why I repeat, people with high blood pressure, heart problems, and expectant mothers, should not take this therapy.

Hot Water Fomentation

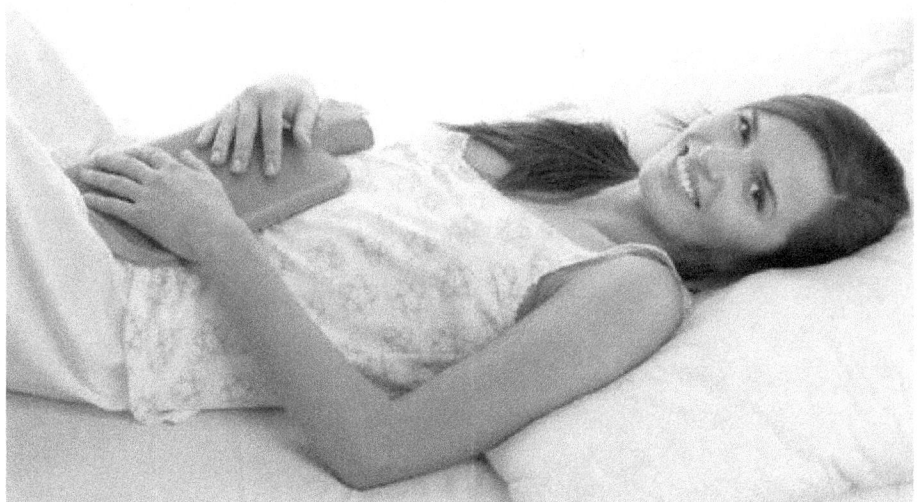

This is the best way in which you can get localized pain relief. Cover the affected region with a hot-water bag or a cloth dipped in hot water. This method of applying heat is going to result in the improvement of circulation and the reduction of pain. That is because the muscles have gotten relaxed.

Remember to wipe the parts subjected to this treatment, with a cloth dipped in cold water, after you have done the fomenting.

Pain relief can take anywhere between 15 minutes to 45 minutes depending on its intensity. You may also need to refill the hot-water bottle with water during the process. Make sure the water is not boiling hot.

Cold water fomentations are also excellent to keep the body cool, especially during summer.

I normally make a cold water foment by filling up my hot-water bottle three fourths with water and put it in the freezer. 4 hours later I have a frozen cold water bottle. Lovely to apply on heated skin, in the summer, especially after a hard day's work outside. Wrap it up in a piece of cloth, so you do not have to bother about the condensation.

Air

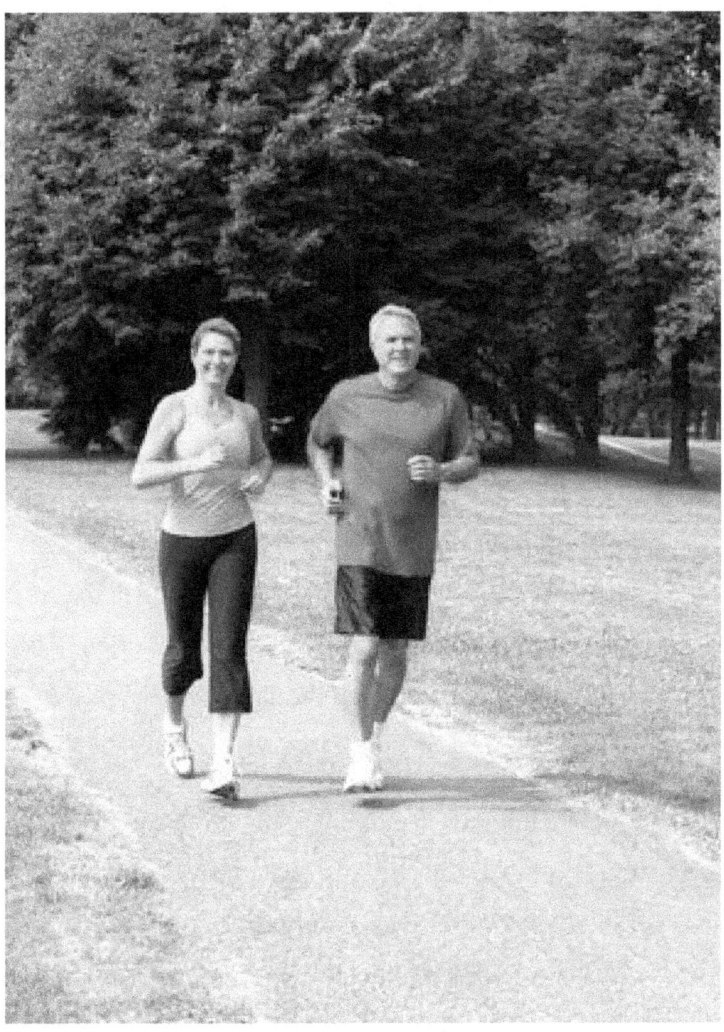

Ah, just enjoying the fresh air...

Air is the 3rd important element of naturopathy. Air therapy or as they say in modern parlance, just getting out of the fug in the room is the best way in which you can get cured of plenty of your diseases and problems.

After you have had a massage, you are going to bake in the sun. That is the sun treatment. You are also going to be breathing in fresh air. That is the a treatment.

In some cases, you may find yourself undergoing the mud bath in the open-air. That is giving you 2 benefits at the same time – Earth and air.

Air therapy is also known as an air bath by naturopaths. Breathing in and breathing out fresh air should be done in wide open spaces, covered with greenery. Accompany this with deep breathing to "aerate" the lungs.

The cool breeze of the early morning, without any vestige of pollution is rich, pure and fresh. It is also full of oxygen. It is going to purify your blood and your body. It is going to feel your mind with good cheer.

Always breathe through your nose when you are walking in the fresh air. This is to filter out any possible particles of dust and pollution. Also, the air is going to get warmed up, when passing through the nasal passages. This is going to have a vigorous effect on your lungs.

Deep breathing is something we have forgotten. Do you know that we are utilizing just a fraction of the capacity of our lungs while breathing? Besides not breathing properly, we were so used in living in the cities are terrified of clogging up our systems with the polluted air. That is why we take shallow breaths.

Deep breathing in an open space, in the greenery is going to eliminate the buildup of carbon dioxide in the body. Shallow breathing means that the carbon dioxide is not eliminated properly from your body. Toxins are thus going to accumulate.

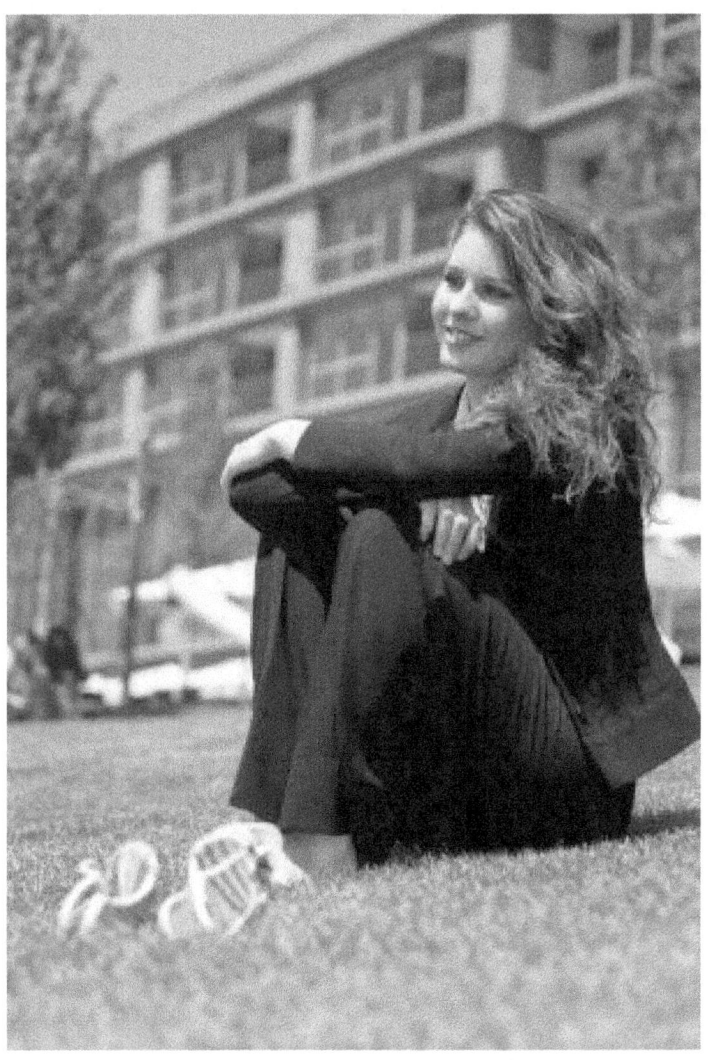

Let nature play her magic on you.

Along with this, make sure that you go to sleep with your face uncovered. The Britishers have a fresh air fetish, that is why it was a running joke that even on the coldest day, they needed a window open. But that was only in Victorian times.

In medieval times, fresh air was considered to be very harmful, and windows were never opened. That is why breathing stale air day in day out, caused so many problems of the lungs and chest.

Even in the winter, make sure that you do not sleep in a closed room. Many of our bedrooms are air-conditioned in the summer. That means we definitely are living in a sterile and stale atmosphere cocooned away from fresh air.

So make sure that there is at least one window open in the winter, to give you a continuous supply of fresh air and getting rid of the stale air accumulating in the room.

Naturally, you are going to be well covered and warm. Try not to sleep in a centrally heated bedroom as far as possible.

Sunlight

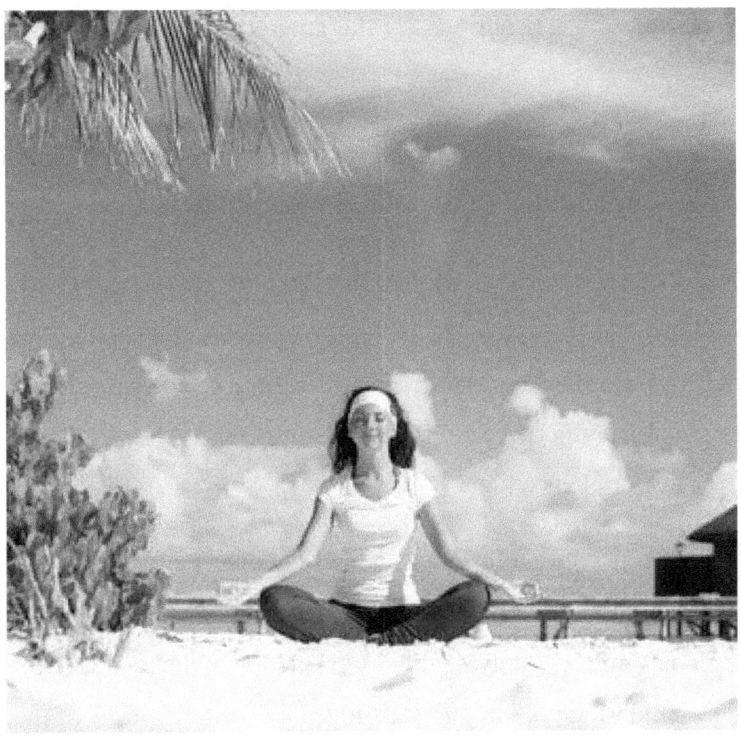

The 4th important factor in helping our body itself is sunlight. Remember that you need about 10 to 15 minutes of exposure to the sun every day in order to keep healthy. But we are so bothered about sunburn and suntan that we do not allow our bodies even the minimal needed access to vitamin D and vitamin B-12.

These 2 vitamins are essential to keep our bodies healthy. Have you heard about the sun worshipers? In all ancient civilizations, the sun was worshiped as one of the most powerful Gods, the giver of light, and the sustainer of life. Today, the word sun worshiping may be associated with all those people tanning themselves on the beach without any sunscreen or protection, and getting badly burned in the hot rays of the sun.

Sunrays are considered to have an invigorating effect on your body. These sunrays, especially at dusk and dawn when the sky turned red were considered to be most beneficial by the ancients, who took "sun baths" at that time.

This Sun Ray assimilation in your body is good for the blood circulation. It relaxes your body and also makes you feel peaceful and serene.

Infrared rays of the sun, especially at dusk and dawn are capable of relaxing and soothing your muscles, reducing swelling and relieving pain. The ultraviolet rays are the important race which produce vitamin D. Stay away from the sun, and you are going to find your bones weakening. You may even suffer from rickets.

This is the reason why children in ancient Greece, Egypt and other ancient Western civilizations were allowed to roam free in the sun, so that their bones could assimilate plenty of vitamin D. Then, at the age of 5, they began to put their childhood behind and start to train as future adults of the country or state.

Ultraviolet rays are essential for good skin. That is why people suffering from skin problems are asked to go out in the sun for at least 2 – 3 minutes. This helps cure the injured skin by killing the bacteria on its surface.

However, in the 21st century, most of us are so scared about sun exposure, because of the fear of diseases caused by the sun that we cover our faces and bodies completely before we go out. And that is why many of us find ourselves suffering from skin diseases.

And we do not realize that a little bit of a sun bath in the morning sun, along with some fresh air would have prevented those pimples and infections.

Sun baths are normally taken in minimal clothing. Cover the head and closed the eyes when you are taking a sun bath. Do not cover your face. Never look directly in the sun. When you are taking a sun bath, choose the miles sunlight in the morning or in the evening. Never take a sun bath in the afternoon, especially when the sun is at its zenith.

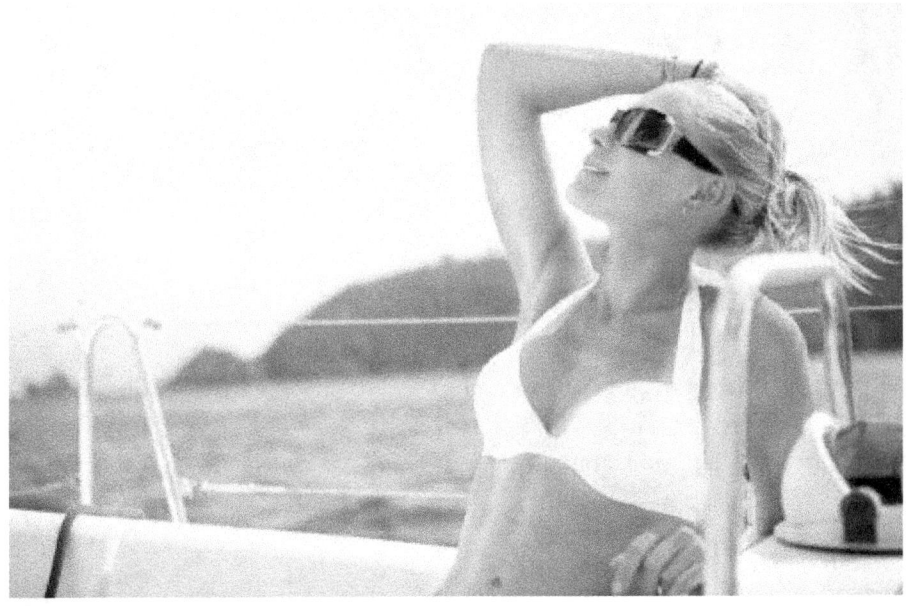

Sun worshiping is all very fine, but a sun bath should never be taken for more than 5 – 10 minutes at a time at the most. Go in into shelter, allow your skin to cool, take some cooling drink and then you can come out again.

Sunlight helps in nourishing your growing muscles. That is the reason why athletes love to bask in the sun. It also improves your resistance power to diseases.

Wounds supposedly healed faster when they were exposed to the sun and fresh air, every ancient warrior knew that. That is why they never bandaged their wounds, as far as possible.

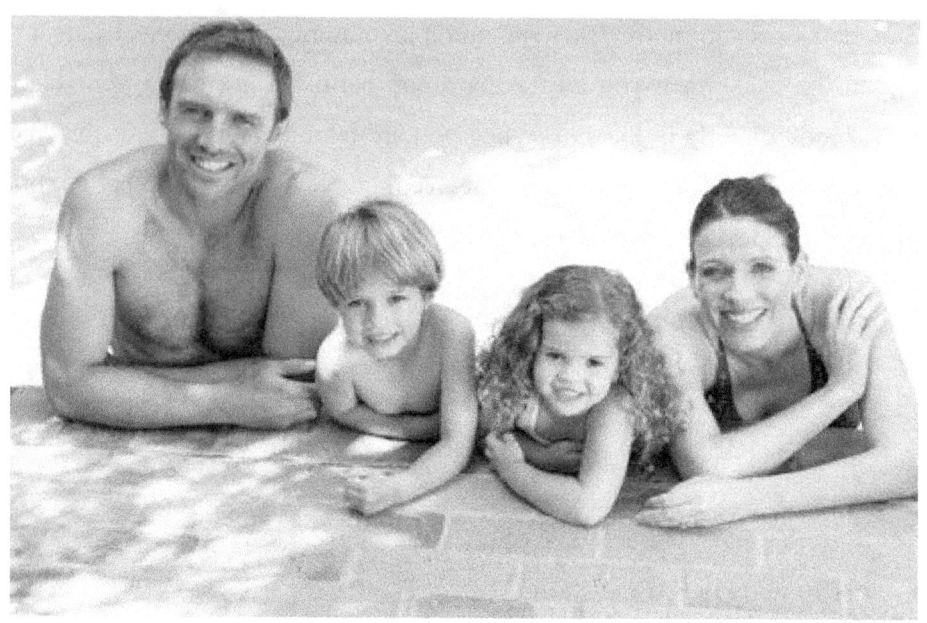

As long as we do not get sunburned…

If a body is undergoing convalescence, he is put out in the sun to relax by his nurse. She knows the efficacy of vitamin D to help heal him and strengthen him.

Believe it or not, cancer is less prevalent in areas where there is plenty of sun throughout the year. Places without sun light shining through the rooms are going to be more prone to disease, because they do not have the natural healing properties of the sun, disinfecting the area.

Start your sun bath by exposing your body to the sunlight for about 5 to 10 minutes. Cover the posterior portion of your body and allow the sun to bathe the anterior part with its healing rays. After 5 minutes, allow the sunrays to play upon the posterior portion of your body.

You can increase the time you spend in the sun, depending on its capacity to bear the sunlight and the heat without getting overly warm or burnt.

If you start feeling giddy, discomfort, or fatigue, that means you have overdone things. Get out of the sun immediately. Also, if you find your skin start to itch or burn, stop your sun bath.

After you have had your sun bath, take a cold water bath. Or you can wipe your body with a piece of cloth wrung out in cold water.

Ether

This is the 5th important as essential element in order to keep yourself healthy and your body to heal itself. Ether means a vacuum. Fasting is a part of the naturopathy treatment given during a therapeutic treatment.

This includes fasting. Fasting here does not mean starving yourself, but not eating a couple of meals once in a while and never missing two meals in a row so that your system gets a chance to get rid of accumulated toxins.

Knowing More about "Fasting"

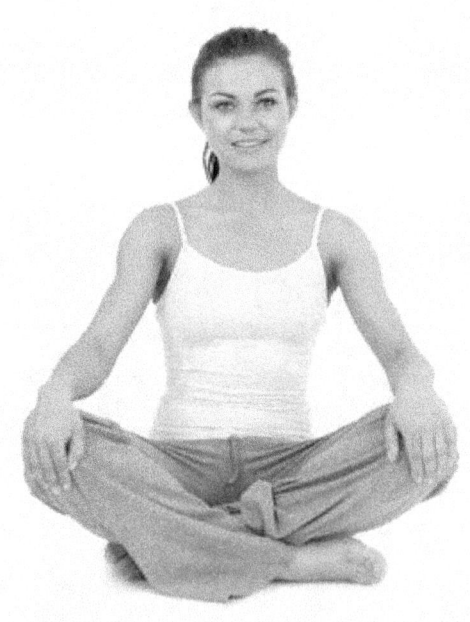

I keep slim and trim by fasting regularly. I skip every 5th and 6th meal, which means I do not eat anything for a major part of every 2nd day.

This is not fasting. This is a potential starvation.

I have noticed that as people grow older, they begin to be more "spiritual" in their outlook, and along with prayers, they begin to "fast" even more. A fast means the total abstinence from eating any kind of food. That means you are not going to take any liquid or solid food, fruit, cereals and water. This is done for a definite period, with a view of giving rest to the different organs of the body, and detoxifying it. This is also supposed to be a purification of the mind, spirit and body.

Is this fasting a healthy activity, you may ask?

Well, I can clearly say that this definitely is not advisable for old people, from a keeping healthy point of view, even though conventional traditionalists, used to fasting, will not agree with me. That is because in plenty of societies all over the world, fasting, at regular periods is a way of life. But then, this does not include eating and drinking absolutely nothing at all throughout the day.

Since ancient times man has been fasting for a number of reasons – both practical and religious. That is why he normally abstained from eating food on a particular day. In olden times, it had nothing to do with religion, but had more to do with whether the hunter of the tribe managed to get a good catch during the day.

If he could not manage to catch anything, the people of the tribe just drank some water, and went off to sleep hungry. This is not "fasting." This is reality brought on by circumstances.

As time went by, people began to abstain from food as a matter of a religious practice, considering it to be a way to achieve some spiritual state of well-being. Priests abstained from food at one meal time or even one day, before the celebration of some holy festival.

Fasting does not mean total abstinence from food. You are going to eat nutritional food items during a fast. Dates are one of them.

This sort of detoxification for just about 8 – 10 hours is acceptable, because your body is not being starved. Remember that your body needs lots of minerals, proteins, carbohydrates, and other essential nutrients in order to function properly. People above the age of 60 cannot afford any sort of malnutrition. They also cannot afford to starve their bodies of these essential nutrients.

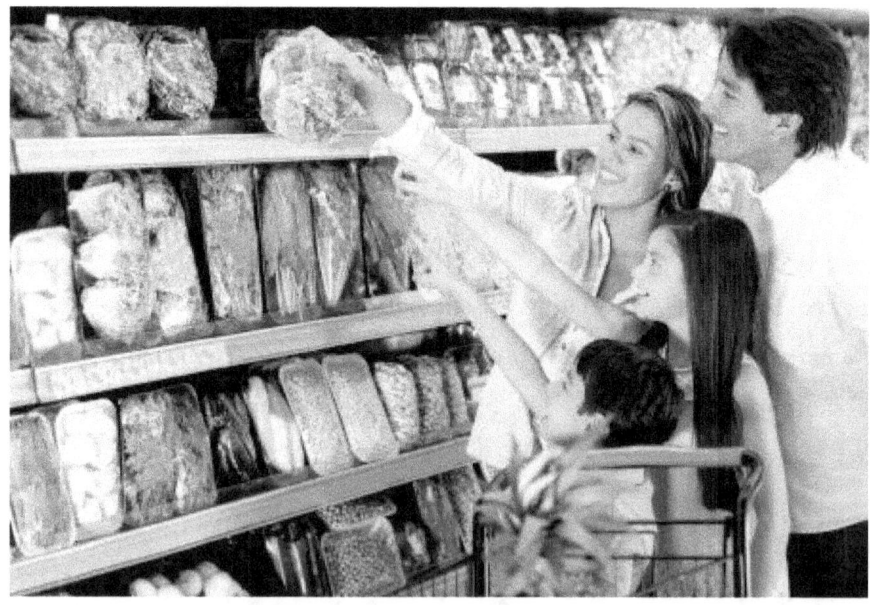

We need all these natural essential nutrients in order to keep healthy

However, if they intend to fast – putting aside any religious significance – the fasting can be done by taking fruit, water or fruit juices. At least the stomach is getting some sort of nutrient and there is no chance of its missing out on liquid intake, which is necessary to keep your body healthy and strong.

Difference between Fasting and Starving Yourself Deliberately

Fasting does not mean starving like I said. Fasting and starving are 2 different conditions. It is true that in both these conditions, you do not eat anything. But fasting is done voluntarily.

Starving is either done due to force of circumstances when you do not have food to eat, or possibly when you are so sick that you cannot manage to eat any food. That means that you are going to suffer from starvation in the long run.

Starving is beyond the control of an individual. When you are sick, your body is going to be using all its power in order to counteract the disease and help heal your body naturally. During this period, your body requires more nourishment, but because it is not functioning normally, you may not feel hungry. But remember that the regular elimination of toxins accumulating in your body needs to take place, whether you are healthy or when you are sick.

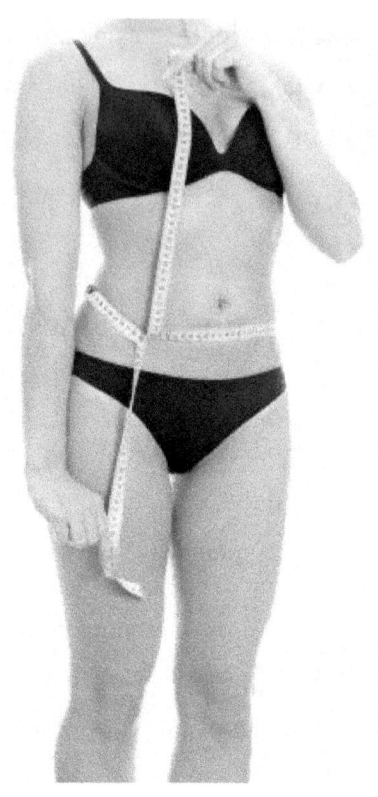

Ooooh, I put on one inch. Fasting for the next 72 hours...

This is definitely not "fasting". It is starvation and your body will not stand it in the long-term. You are soon going to suffer from malnutrition and eating disorders.

When your body does not need any nourishment, and your appetite is dormant, any sort of abstention from eating can be considered to be fasting. Remember that your body requires heat and fuel, even while you are fasting. That is when your body begins to burn all the "fuel", already present in it to keep it functioning normally, because it knows that it is not going to have food coming in soon.

Starvation is going to be the condition in which your cells and organs are slowly going to deteriorate because of continuous fasting. If you have been fasting over a long period of time, you are going to find yourself starving and suffering from malnutrition.

Fasting in order to lose weight is the new 21st-century fad. And that is why many people suffer from eating disorders, because firstly, they are depriving their body of the essential natural nutrients required to keep healthy. They may lose weight temporarily, but that is because the body has got rid of the accumulated toxins. But all that weight is going to come back again, as soon as they start eating again.

An old person cannot afford to have the essential stored fuel in his body "burned" up, because he is not eating. This burning process includes the catabolism of fat and blood sugar. If the fastest continued after all the present body fat is used up, the fibers and the cells of your organs are going to disintegrate and a desperate body is going to derive its nourishment from them. This is definitely harmful and potentially dangerous.

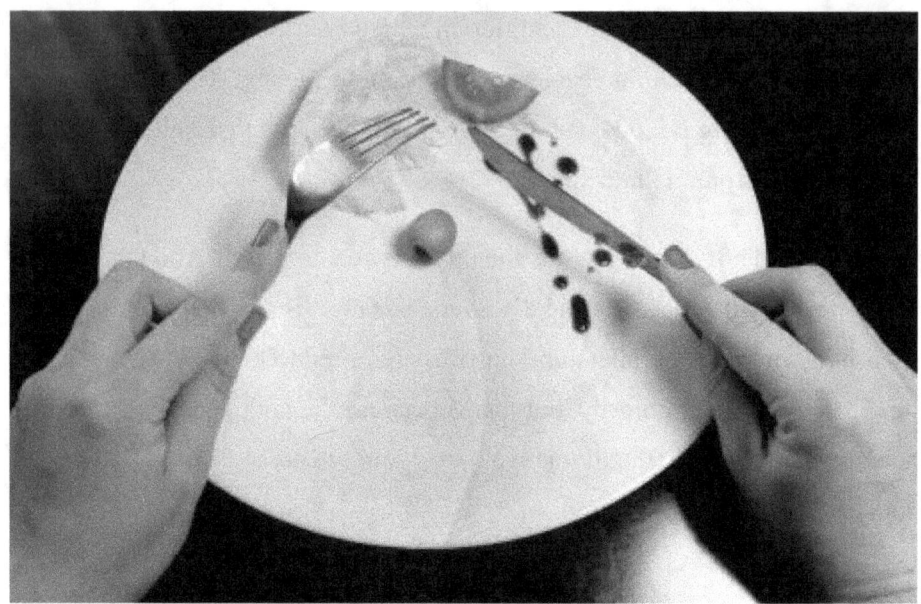

Why would any sane, normal and healthy person want to starve oneself on purpose for long periods of time, when she or he has plenty of access to food? All under the polite garb of "fasting" or dieting when actually they are starving themselves?

A majority of people nowadays "fast" for anywhere between 9 to 10 days to one month, for a number of reasons, including possible spiritual progress and mental peace. But this fasting process does not mean that they deprive their body of essential nutrients. The body is fed fruit juices, fresh fruit, and other fast related foods, which means that the system is still working in a healthy fashion, even though the diet has changed.

Simple, light and nutritious food should be taken for the period of the fast. Raw vegetables, sprouted cereals, and sprouted pulses should be taken in large quantities so that your body is not deprived of minerals and vitamins needed to detoxify it.

In addition to this, the surplus vitamins and nutrients are stored away in the body, to be used at will, if the person is determined to extend his fasting period.

At the time of ending the fast you need to end it with a little quantity of orange juice or lemon juice. That is because the digestive system has been comparatively inactive during this period. The intestines may have shrunk in size, if the fasting was done over a longer period of time.

So great care needs to be taken before burdening these "dormant" digestive organs, with a heavy meal. For the first couple of days, drink just fruit juices. After 4 – 5 days, you can take boiled vegetables and cooked food should be given after a week or so.

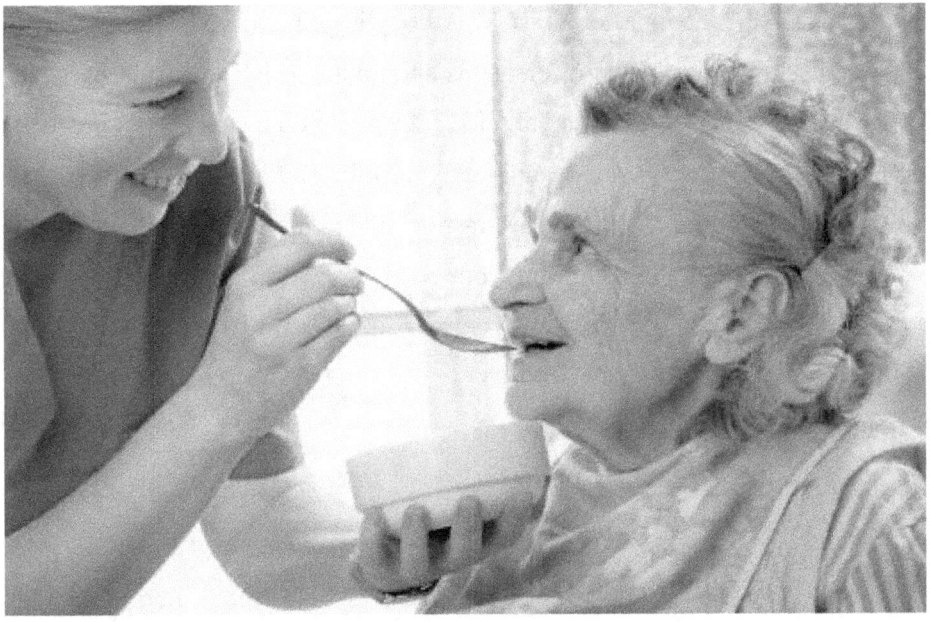

Old people should never be allowed to fast, because any sort of abstinence from meals is going to have a detrimental effect on their naturally weakening bodies.

If they persist on fasting due to religious and spiritual beliefs, feed them plenty of fruit and vegetables. Make sure that they have some sort of cooked food at least once a day. This is going to prevent their intestines from "shrinking".

Giving them lots of rich and fatty food in the hope that they are going to regain their energy and weight lost during a fast is dangerous and foolish.

Remember that the necessity of fasting is going to arise only when you have not bothered much about regular meals, proper diet, and proportion of diet when you eat and drink. You can go through a lifetime without fasting, if you have followed "proper eating" rules throughout your life.

The fasting process is done to detoxify your body. The moment you start eating a rich diet again after a fast, your body is going to become a storehouse of these poisonous elements and toxins which cause diseases, yet once again. You can miss a meal once a week, if you have been eating regular meals 3 times a day throughout your life. But missing meals regularly, and thinking that you are fasting, and you are thus losing weight is misleading. You are just harming your body.

Conclusion

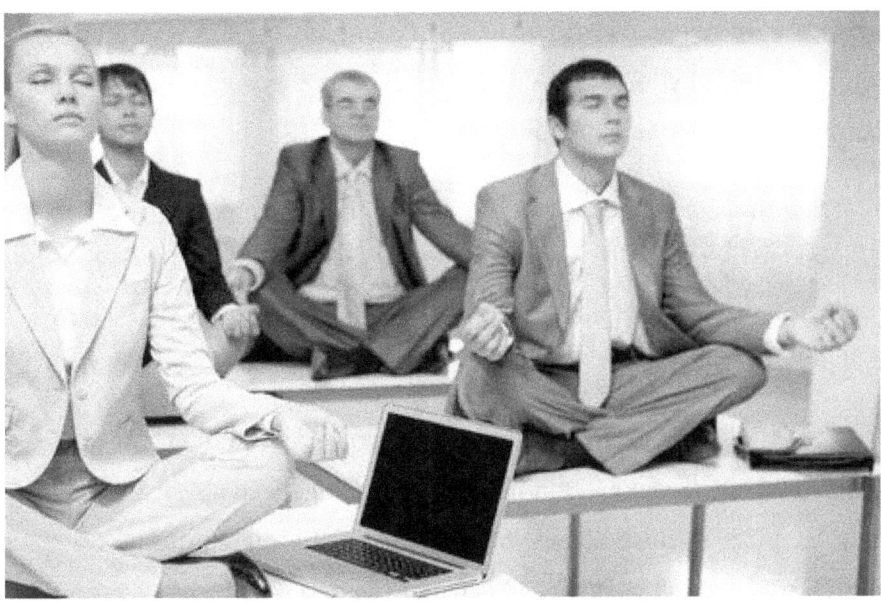

Meditation is one way in which your body can relax and your mind can grow tension free and stress-free.

This book has given you lots of information on how you can let your body heal itself naturally. All the methods given here are time tested and have been very effective in helping one cure oneself in the most natural and beneficial way possible.

Meditation, sun baths, massages, mud packs, yoga, simple, and nutritious food, complete and partial fasting with a water or food diet, hydrotherapy, and other methods are used to help heal your body naturally. Naturopaths do not treat infectious diseases. Diet plays a very important role in healing along with other therapies.

As you going to detoxification mode, naturopaths are going to advise boiled, steamed and bland food all the while you are undergoing therapy. That is because all the methods used to detoxify your body cannot work to their optimum limit, if you keep stuffing yourself with foods which cause more toxins to be created in your body.

So if you find yourself eating plenty of fruit and vegetables, and not being allowed meat products, fatty and spicy products during a healing process, take a deep breath and tell yourself – it is for my own good. My body is healing itself.

To aid healing, the ancients also advocated prayer. According to them, spiritual healing, went hand-in-hand with emotional and physical healing. Also, exercise, meditation and yoga were parts of healing therapy. The main priority was to think positive and get your mind to your body.

And then the body did the rest, with a little bit of assistance from nature.

So learn to let your body heal itself. Live Long and Prosper!

Author Bio

Dueep Jyot Singh is a Management and IT Professional who managed to gather Postgraduate qualifications in Management and English and Degrees in Science, French and Education while pursuing different enjoyable career options like being an hospital administrator, IT,SEO and HRD Database Manager/ trainer, movie , radio and TV scriptwriter, theatre artiste and public speaker, lecturer in French, Marketing and Advertising, ex-Editor of Hearts On Fire (now known as Solstice) Books Missouri USA, advice columnist and cartoonist, publisher and Aviation School trainer, ex-moderator on Medico.in, banker, student councilor ,travelogue writer … among other things!

One fine morning, she decided that she had enough of killing herself by Degrees and went back to her first love -- writing. It's more enjoyable! She already has 48 published academic and 14 fiction- in- different- genre books under her belt.

When she is not designing websites or making Graphic design illustrations for clients , she is browsing through old bookshops hunting for treasures, of which she has an enviable collection – including R.L. Stevenson, O.Henry, Dornford Yates, Maurice Walsh, De Maupassant, Victor Hugo, Sapper, C.N. Williamson, "Bartimeus" and the crown of her collection- Dickens "The Old Curiosity Shop," and so on… Just call her "Renaissance Woman") - collecting herbal remedies, acting like Universal Helping Hand/Agony Aunt, or escaping to her dear mountains for a bit of exploring, collecting herbs and plants and trekking.

Check out some of the other JD-Biz Publishing books

Gardening Series on Amazon

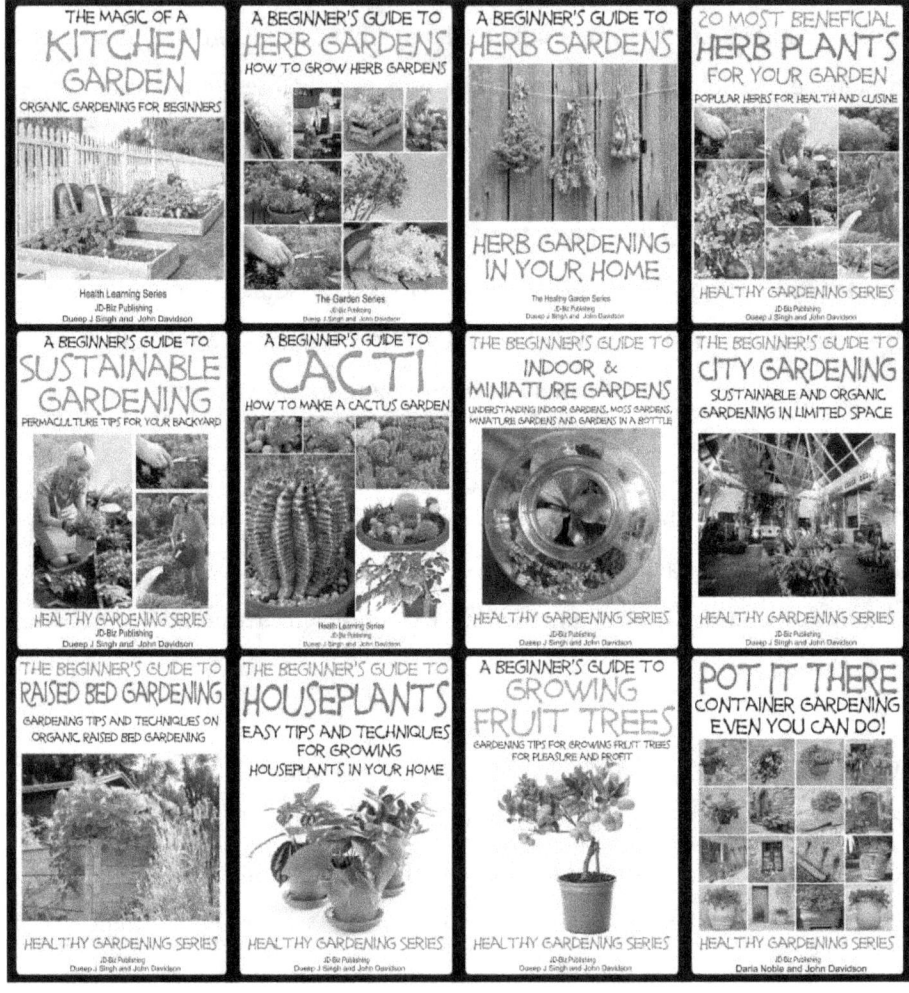

Health Learning Series

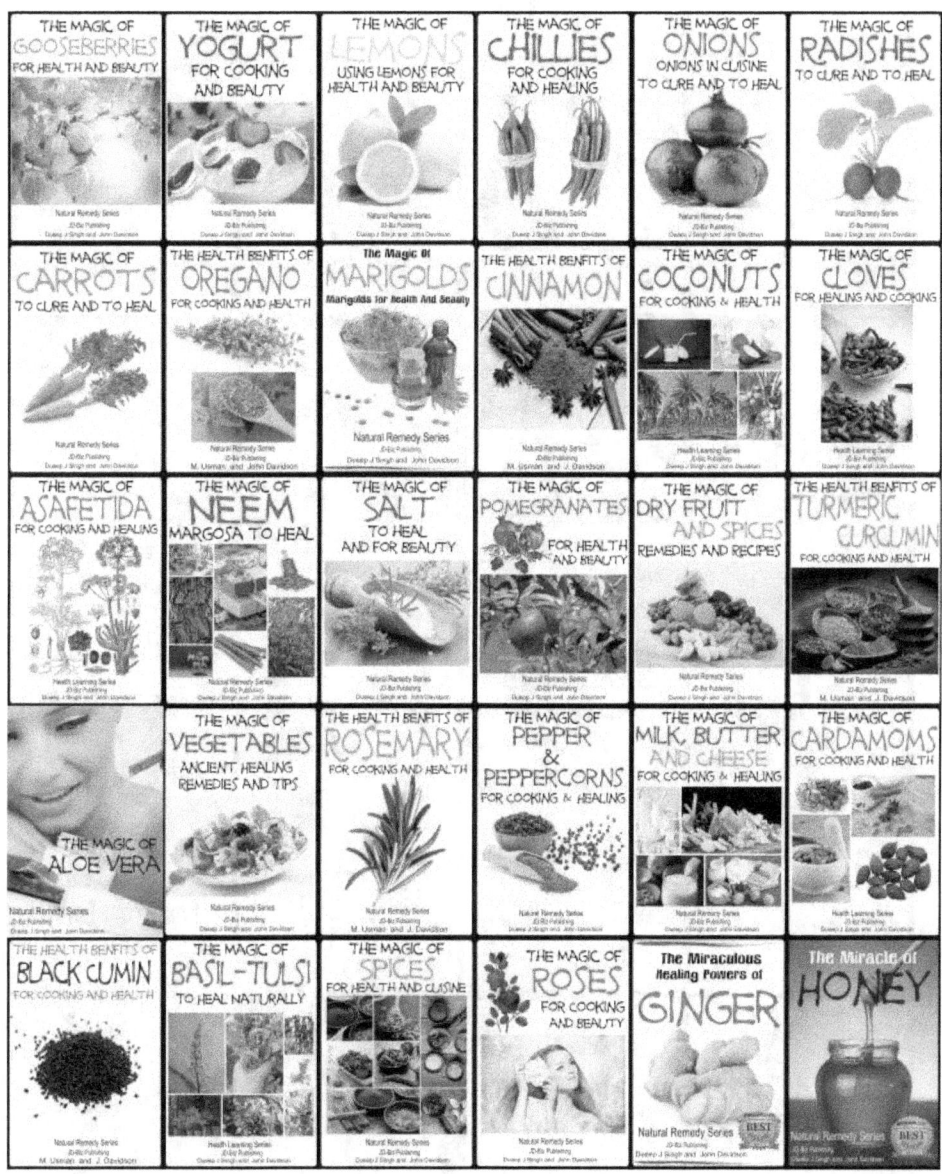

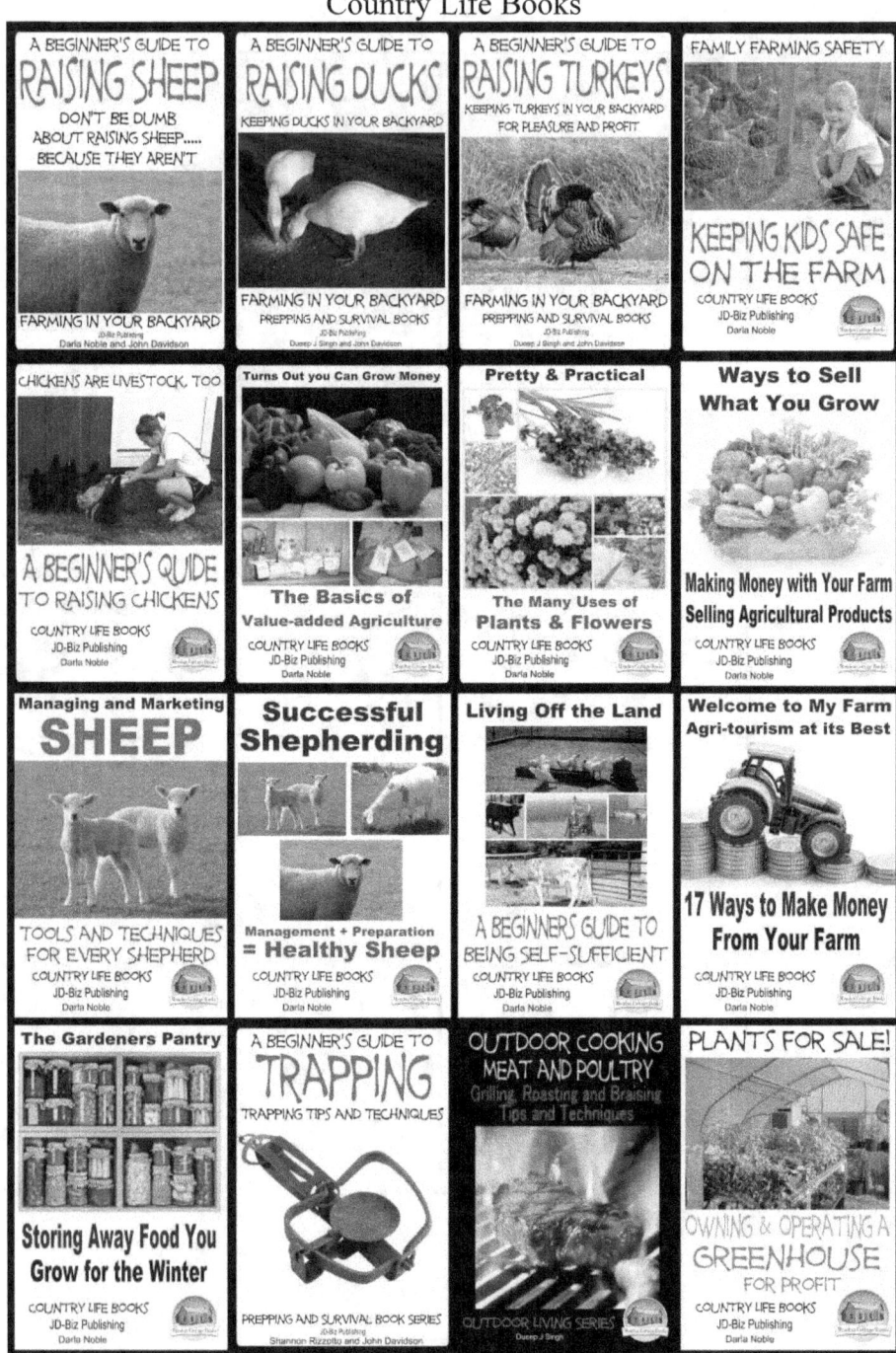

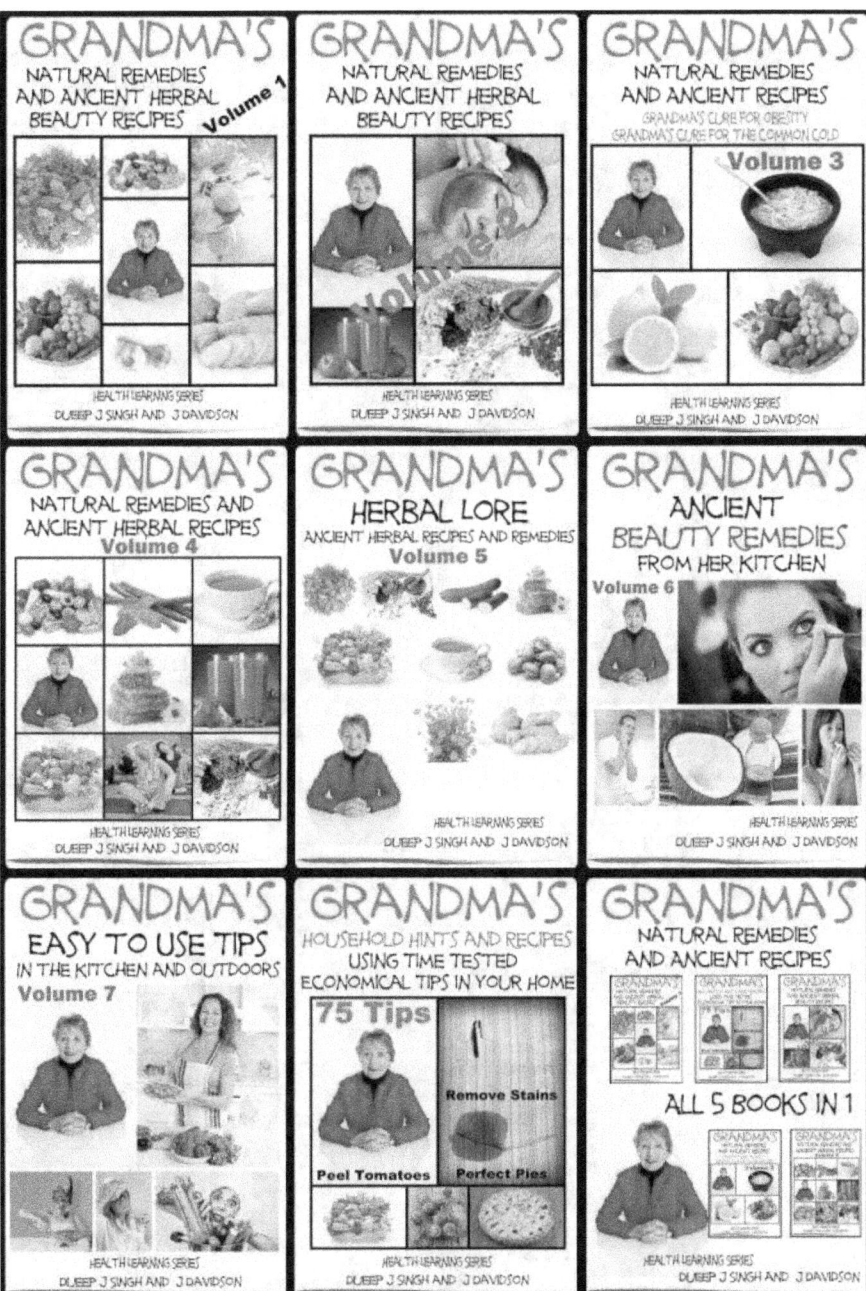

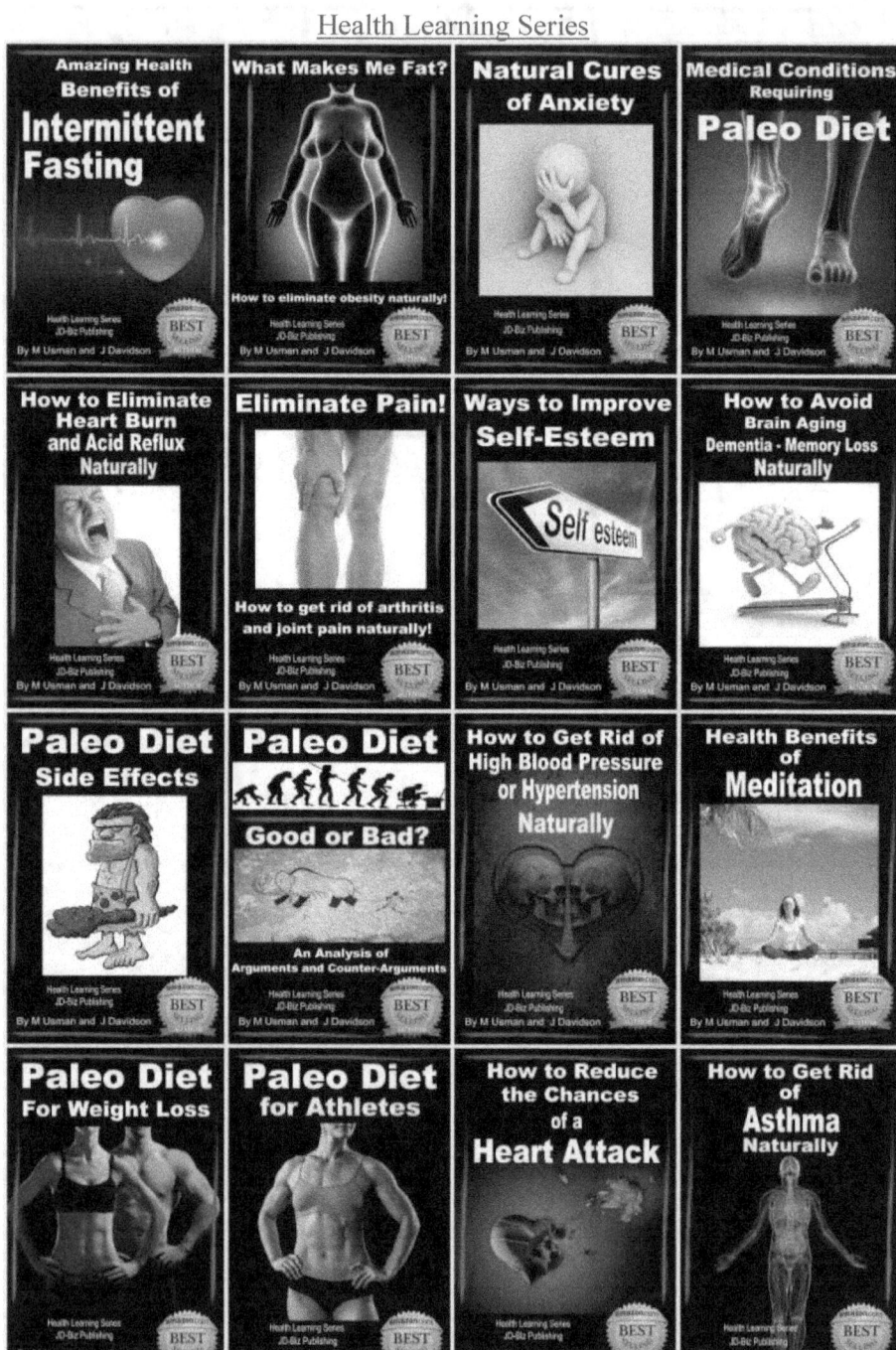

Amazing Animal Book Series

Learn To Draw Series

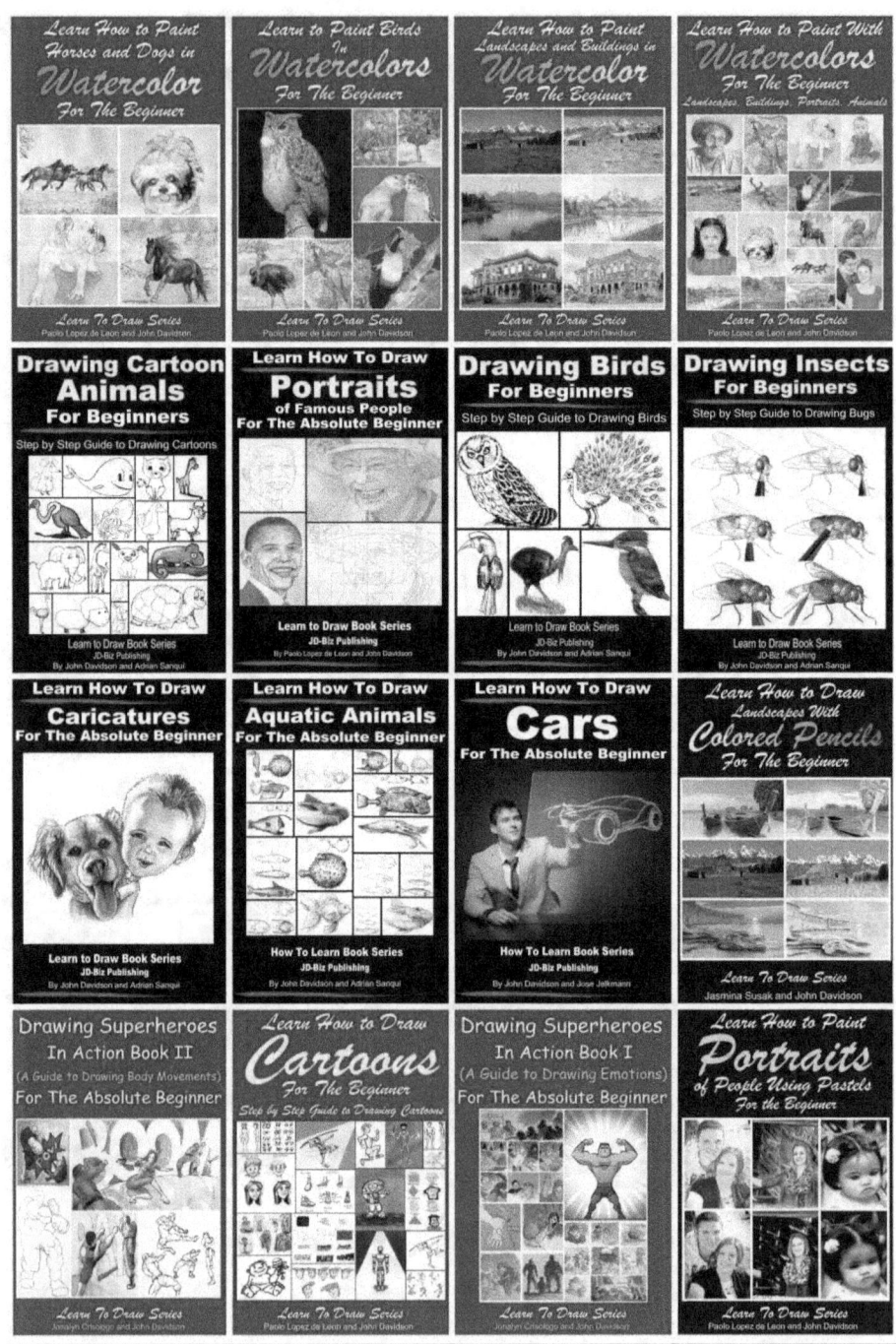

How to Build and Plan Books

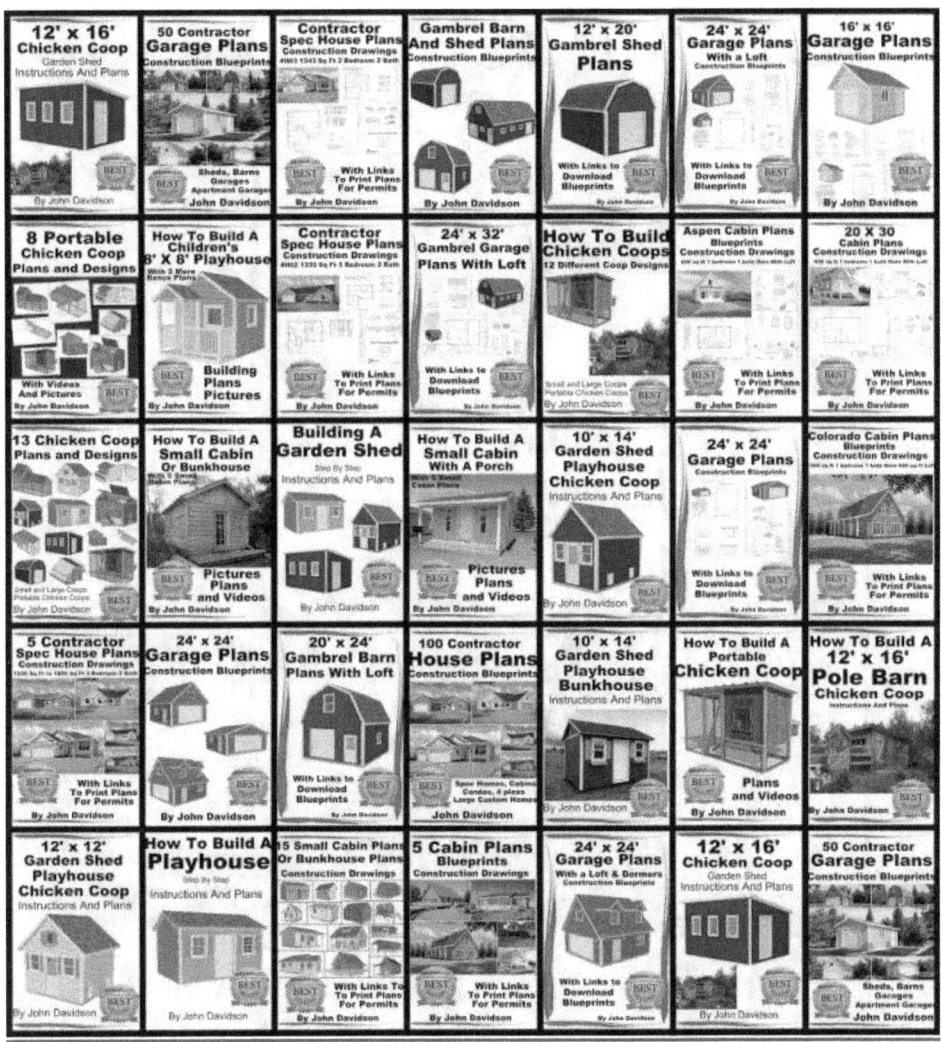

Entrepreneur Book Series

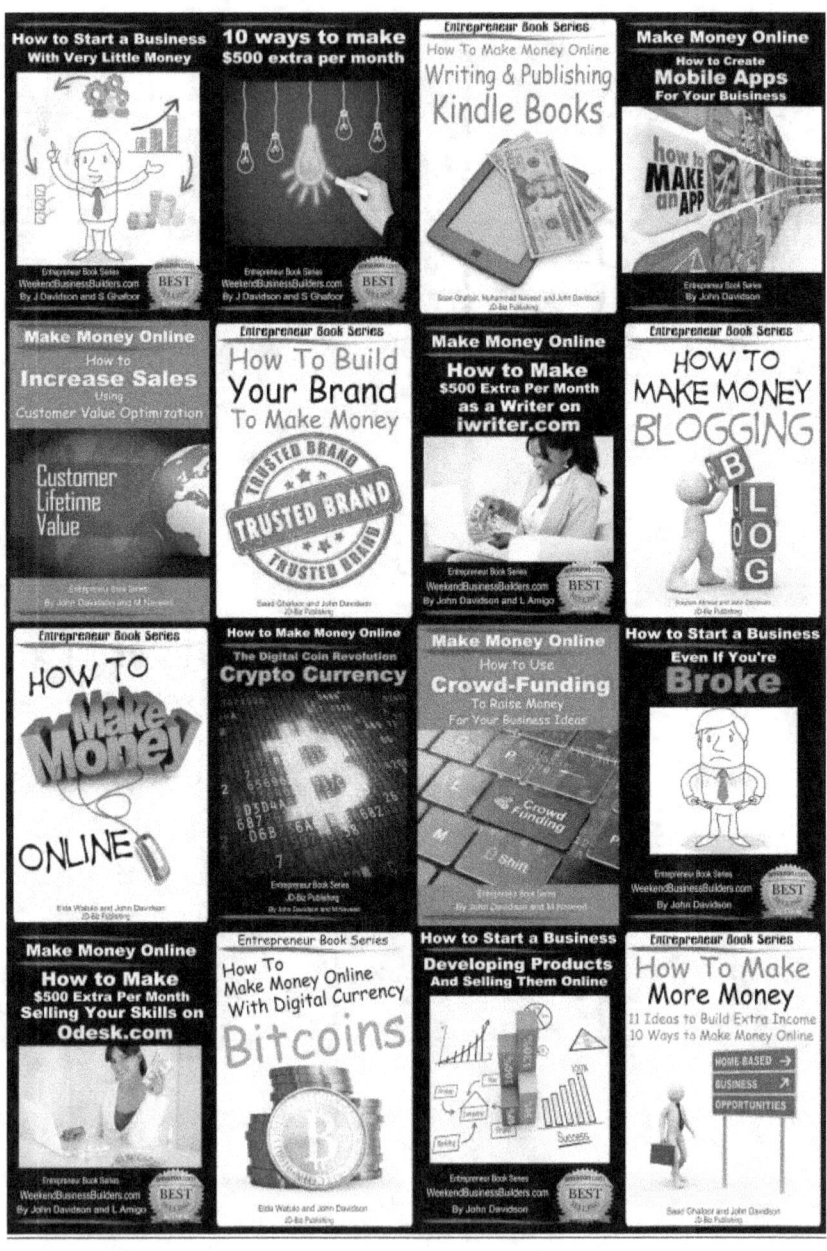

Our books are available at

1. Amazon.com

2. Barnes and Noble

3. Itunes

4. Kobo

5. Smashwords

6. Google Play Books

Publisher

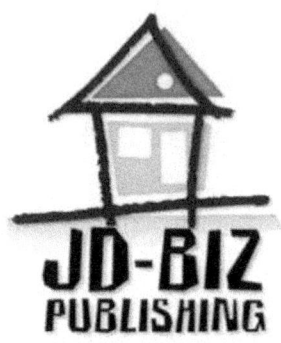

JD-Biz Corp

P O Box 374

Mendon, Utah 84325

http://www.jd-biz.com/

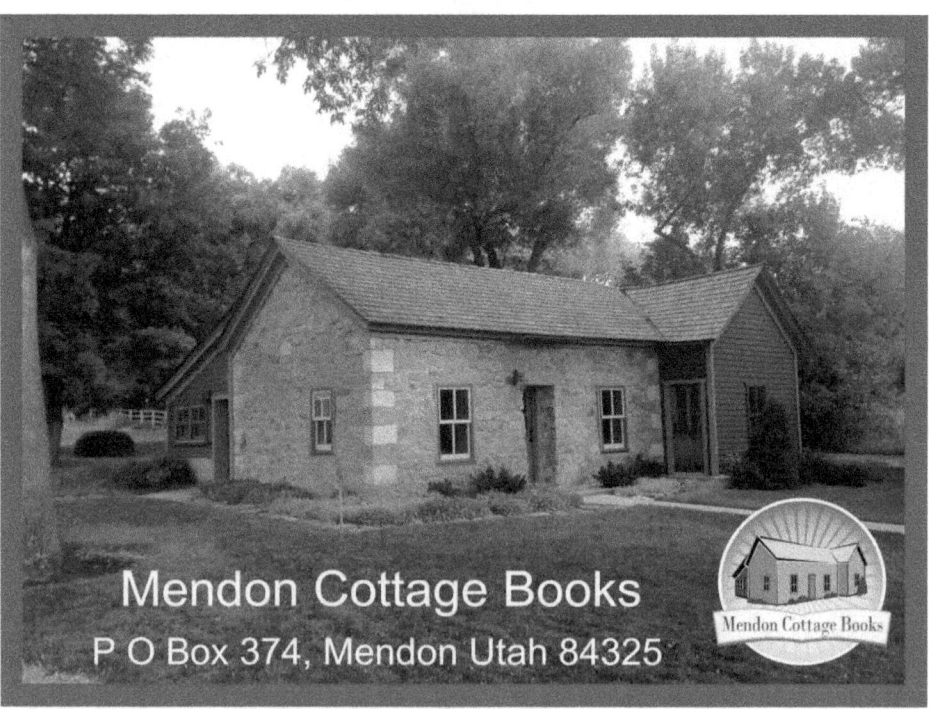

Mendon Cottage Books

P O Box 374, Mendon Utah 84325